The Nurse Mentor and Reviewer Update Book

The Nurse Mentor and Reviewer Update Book

**Edited by
Cyril Murray, Lyn Rosen and
Karen Staniland**

 Open University Press

Open University Press
McGraw-Hill Education
McGraw-Hill House
Shoppenhangers Road
Maidenhead
Berkshire
England
SL6 2QL

email: enquiries@openup.co.uk
world wide web: http://www.openup.co.uk

and Two Penn Plaza, New York, NY 10121-2289, USA

First published 2010

A catalogue record of this book is available from the British Library

ISBN-13: 978–0–335–24119–4
ISBN-10: 0335241190

Library of Congress Cataloging-in-Publication Data
CIP data applied for

Typeset by RefineCatch Limited, Bungay, Suffolk
Printed in the UK by Bell and Bain Ltd, Glasgow

Mixed Sources
Product group from well-managed
forests and other controlled sources
www.fsc.org Cert no. TT-COC-002769
© 1996 Forest Stewardship Council

FSC

The *McGraw·Hill* Companies

Contents

About the Editors and Contributors

Mary R. Douglas MSc Health Services Research, BSc(H), RGN, Head of Learning and Development at Salford Royal NHS Foundation Trust, Salford. Mary leads on supporting the breadth of the student experience and ensuring the provision of high quality multi-professional clinical learning environments. Her research interests include patient-centred built healthcare environments and professional practice developments.

Cyril Murray MSc, BA, DipN (London), CertEd, RN, RCNT, RNT, FETC, GICC 100. Worked as a Senior Lecturer at the University of Salford before retiring in July 2009. Cyril held a number of senior educational posts over the last 20 years including partnerships and collaboration between higher education and practice, academic enterprise, staff development and international lead link. He has a keen interest in professional development particularly mentorship and enhancement of the student learning experience in clinical practice.

Lyn Rosen BSc(H), RN, RM, CertEd, RCNT. Lecturer, School of Nursing, Faculty of Health and Social Care, University of Salford. Lyn is involved in the promotion of flexible learning and e-learning. She has a special interest in promoting work-based learning as a discipline in its own right, both as a curriculum component and as part of professional development in the clinical environment.

Karen Staniland PhD, MSc, BSc(H), CertEd, RCNT, DipN (London), RN, RM. Senior Lecturer, School of Nursing, Faculty of Health and Social Care, University of Salford. Karen is involved with the promotion of flexible, work-based learning and e-learning in nursing. Her main research interest lies in healthcare quality improvement at the bedside in relation to clinical governance and the essence of care.

Preface

Many books have been written about teaching and learning but there has never been a text written specifically for **mentors** and their **reviewers/ appraisers**.

So how will you know if this book is for you? Well you can start by asking yourself the following questions:

- Are you a qualified mentor or aspiring to become one?
- Are you a qualified mentor but unsure of the activities to undertake or the evidence which should be produced to demonstrate evidence of **annual updating** in your work to your employer?
- Are you a nurse manager or reviewer/appraiser of mentors who would benefit from guidance on how judgements can be made about the evidence mentors may produce to demonstrate their competence to remain on the live mentor register?

If you answered *yes* to one or more of these questions then this book is *definitely* for you.

However, this book has a broader applicability as it is relevant to all professional nurses on the Nursing and Midwifery Council (NMC) professional register who wish to develop their knowledge and understanding on how to support and facilitate the development of other learners. Furthermore, those nurses who fulfil educator roles will find this book a useful resource to support mentors and other nurses in professional updating activities and/or facilitating the development of student learning. The style of presentation can be adapted to the professional role and work context of each reader.

Concerns about the practices of mentors

As you may know, the NMC as a regulatory body sets policies and standards in order to protect the public and direct the professional body of practitioners. Concerns have been raised that nurses functioning as mentors have not been fulfilling their professional responsibilities as accountable practitioners by 'failing to fail' students (Duffy 2003). Furthermore, attendances at annual updating activities to keep abreast of educational developments in order to fulfil this role have been poor. The pressures of patient care are frequently cited as taking priority over mentor updating, in addition to staff shortages and a lack of information about the actual provision of updates (Pulsford *et al.* 2002; McVeigh *et al.* 2009).

The release of the **NMC Standards** (NMC 2006, 2008) addresses these short-falls, as it clearly articulates the professional **accountability** and responsibilities of both mentors and their employers with regard to mentorship. Mentors have to demonstrate ongoing competence through evidence of annual updating activities in order to remain on the live mentor register (held by their employer). They will be subject to a review every three years linked to their appraisal scheme. Employers will need to develop systems which dovetail the professional body requirements with the contractual responsibilities on how practitioners fulfil their job role.

How can this book help you?

This book offers a timely, flexible, alternative practical resource to meet the evidence requirements of an annual mandatory update for mentors in order to meet the NMC standards (2008). It can be utilized at a time, place and pace set by you and will help you overcome some of the current constraints on attending updating events. It will also assist the appraiser/reviewer in judging the nature and evidence of the updating activities and application by the mentor within the job role.

The book is intended to be a realistic activity book which includes a number of case studies that can be worked through individually or with other professionals. The case studies can be assessed and marked as the answers are provided. They are problem-based situations that have actually arisen in practice and promote the **reliability** and transfer of knowledge and skills into practice.

Alternatively, the book could also double up as a teaching or resource aid for nurse educators whose responsibilities include the updating of mentors.

What does each chapter contain?

Chapter 1 will provide the foundations and framework for the focus and content of the rest of the book. It will begin by outlining the history of mentorship and then focus more specifically on literature within nursing in the United Kingdom. Some of the ambiguities that have arisen in the usage of such a term and the conflicts that may potentially arise in practice will be presented. This background information will provide the foundation for understanding the current Nursing and Midwifery Council's requirements for mentors which is documented in the standard to 'support learning and assessment in practice' (NMC 2008). This standard has made significant changes to the professional responsibilities of both individual practitioners and their employers for future mentorship activities.

The concept of 'competence' will form the nucleus of **Chapter 2** as the literature offers many ambiguous and confusing definitions of the word. Two perspectives will be presented in which competence is viewed as a description, or action or outcome of performance which is observed in practice, versus the view that competence is associated with a cluster of attributes and abilities (critical thinking, problem solving etc.) that are essential to performance. Whilst both perspectives may have critics they provide a useful starting point to the analysis on how to measure competence. In addition they provide an analysis of the civil 'standard of proof' which is used by the NMC in professional regulatory hearings in which judgements about competence and fitness to practice may occur. The chapter concludes with an outline of how ongoing competence as a mentor could be linked to an employer-led appraisal system incorporating the National Health Service (NHS) Knowledge and Skills Framework (DH 2004).

Chapter 3 will present a perspective on the operational system and structure which healthcare organizations may consider when addressing the ongoing competence of mentors by reviewers. Employer-led appraisal schemes involve the assessment and judgement of the types and quality of evidence mentors present to demonstrate how ongoing competence has been maintained. This chapter will explore how appraisers/reviewers analyse this evidence to determine whether mentors should be added or removed from the live register. The chapter will then build on the first two chapters by addressing the role of the **reviewer** (a reviewer may be a manager or another healthcare practitioner as determined locally) in the appraisal process. No academic levels will be presented within this book, as judgements about how ongoing competence is applied within the job role must be linked to employer-led appraisal systems (NMC 2008), which are locally designed and determined.

Throughout the book emphasis will be placed upon promoting and maintaining ongoing competence. There are many different approaches to this and **Chapter 4** utilizes a case study approach in exploring each of the eight NMC standards. Specifically, mentors can work through a series of questions relating to a scenario (that is a 'real' issue associated with mentoring) to develop their ongoing knowledge and skills. This can then be applied in their professional practice from which evidence can be produced to demonstrate their ongoing competence and meet the requirements for their employer-led appraisal system. Issues such as ethics, special needs, leadership etc. are incorporated within the unique design feature of these case studies.

There are many ways in which mentors can update which are not solely restricted to attendance at events organized by **higher education institutions**.

Chapter 5 outlines a range of activities (of which **case studies** form but one solution as demonstrated in Chapter 4) which could be undertaken on an annual basis to support a mentor's updating and professional development. The demonstration of ongoing competence must become an integral part of a mentor's existing role and can be achieved by incorporating a range of the activities presented in this chapter.

The chapter consists of a range of practical activities which link the role of mentors to the job requirements within their work role and the appraisal system which will review this. A step-by-step approach linked to the NHS KSF (DH 2004) **review process** will be outlined, culminating in a list of possible sources of **evidence** which mentors could generate to demonstrate their ongoing competence. This information will be useful for reviewers as well as mentors.

References

DH (Department of Health) (2004) *The NHS Knowledge and Skills Framework and Development Review Process*. London: Department of Health.

Duffy, K. (2003) *Failing Students: A Qualitative Study of Factors that Influence the Decisions Regarding Assessment of Students' Competence in Practice*. London: NMC.

McVeigh, H., Ford, K., O'Donnell, A., Rushby, C. and Squance, J. (2009) A framework for mentor support in community-based placements, *Nursing Standard*, 23 (45): 35–41.

NMC (Nursing and Midwifery Council) (2006) *Standards to Support Learning and Assessment in Practice*. London: NMC.

NMC (2008) *Standards to Support Learning and Assessment in Practice*. London: NMC.

Pulsford, D., Boit, K. and Owen, S. (2002) Are mentors ready to make a difference? A survey of mentors' attitudes towards nurse education, *Nurse Education Today*, 22: 439–46.

Acknowledgements

We would like to thank the Nursing and Midwifery Council for providing permission to reproduce material for this book from their standards, policies and circulars. Every effort has been made to trace and acknowledge ownership of copyright from all other material reproduced in this book. The publishers will be pleased to make suitable arrangements to clear permission with any copyright holders whom it has not been possible to contact.

We would also like to acknowledge the contributions of Natalie Yates Bolton, Julia Cappleman, Elizabeth Charnock, Dawn Gawthorpe, Annabella Gloster, Dawn Hennefer, Kate Hodginson, Jane Jenkins and Raymond Stansfield who work as academic staff within the University of Salford and assisted with the production of the materials for some of the case studies.

Praise for this book

This is an innovative book which takes account of the professional development of the qualified nurse as it relates to their specific role as a mentor. Of particular value is the way in which the theory and practice have been integrated throughout and in particular the focus on accountability issues of the mentor role in protection of the public and their gatekeeper role to the profession. The case studies and possible responses by the reader provide an excellent framework for the individual and their development in the role, whilst the links to the Knowledge Skills Framework (KSF) will be invaluable to those appraisers and professional development departments in health care organisations. An excellent foundation text for practitioners who wish to undertake the mentor role and for developing the skills of those already undertaking the role and wish to be updated and enhance their knowledge and practice.

Karen Holland, Research Fellow, University of Salford, UK
and Editor, *Nurse Education in Practice*

Part 1

Mentorship, Competence and Placement Provider Responsibilities

1

Mentorship: Past, Present and Future

Cyril Murray and Karen Staniland

Aim

The aim of this chapter will be to provide a review of mentorship within a United Kingdom context.

Learning outcomes

After reading this chapter you will be able to:

- outline the history of mentorship;
- identify the Nursing and Midwifery Council's requirements for practitioners undertaking the role as a mentor;
- discuss how ongoing competence is necessary for practitioners to remain on the live mentor register.

This chapter will begin by briefly outlining the history of mentorship and will then focus more specifically on the literature within nursing in the United Kingdom. In doing this we will consider some of the ambiguities that have arisen in the usage of such a term and present the current definition and role of the mentor in accordance with the NMC's standards. However, it is not the intention to give a full history of mentorship here and readers are advised to use the relevant references for further detail.

The key elements of the NMC standards will be summarized. From this you will be able to identify the knowledge and skills which you as a mentor need to apply in practice to support and assess students and what is required to demonstrate your ongoing competence to continue fulfilling this important professional role.

The history of mentorship

Where did the concept of 'mentorship' originate from?

The concept of mentorship is said to have its origins in Homer's Odyssey in the form of Mentor, who brought up Odysseus's son Telemachaus when he was absent (Bracken and Davis 1989; Donovan 1990; Barlow 1991). A mentor in this context is portrayed as a trusted and older wise friend who takes on the responsibility for the learning and development of a younger man in the absence of a parent (Maggs 1994; Andrews 1999). Modern 'genesis' of the mentorship term can, however, be related to North American businesses and the feminist movement of the 1960s (Maggs 1994: 24). Clutterbuck (1985) and Morris *et al.* (1988) also suggest that mentorship has an alliance with the guilds master–apprenticeship model of instruction and mastery (WNB 1992) and Myrick (1988) pointed out an association to Florence Nightingale (Maggs 1994).

Whilst the term mentorship has traditionally been associated with the medical, law and business professions, early literature on the idea began to appear in the nursing and midwifery literature in the 1960s and was generally of North American origin (Maggs 1994). Literature in the UK then began to identify ambiguities in the term and perception of 'mentorship', and the lack of empirical evidence for the success of such a role (Shamian and Lemieux 1984; Shamian and Inhaber 1985; Myrick 1988; Foy and Waltho 1989). Literature in the 1990s was concerned with the definition of the concept, determining what the role entailed and highlighting the lack of agreement as to what mentorship actually was (Donovan 1990; Morle 1990; Armitage and Burnard 1991; Anforth 1992; Jinks and Williams 1994; Neary *et al.* 1994; Andrews 1999).

When was mentorship incorporated into pre-registration programmes?

Clinical learning in nurse training programmes has been customarily associated with the model of apprenticeship where students learnt but, more importantly, also provided a service in clinical practice. In this respect student learning in practice was given less attention than the service aspect of 'getting the work done' (Melia 1987). The introduction of Project 2000 programmes was revolutionary in changing this as students' learning needs took precedence over service contribution. Students gained supernumerary status for a large proportion of their programme and it seemed logical therefore that some formal recognition for the supervision of these supernumerary students be introduced.

Informal mentoring took place before Project 2000 to a certain degree but with the introduction of Project 2000, formal mentorship programmes became integral to pre-registration education in the late 1990s (Andrews 1999). Consequently, since 1997 all nursing students in training should have experienced some form of formal mentoring.

Confusion about the actual role of the mentor

It is important to acknowledge and be aware that whilst these changes were occurring there was a continuing debate concerning the elusive definition of the role and function of a mentor in nursing, as this has caused some conflict in practice. Whilst the English National Board (ENB 1987) initially made reference to mentors as 'wise reliable counsellors' and 'trusted advisers' which mirrored traditional thinking, other facets of the expected role of a mentor in nursing were incompatible with this position, such as undertaking a role involving 'supervision and assessment' (ENB 1988). This caused confusion and a lack of clarity for mentors and nurse educators. Neary *et al.* (1994) clearly identified the interchangeable uses of the terms depicting the mentor role as co-ordinator, practice facilitator and preceptor whilst Wilson-Barnett *et al.* (1995) added those of mentor, assessor and supervisor.

To help clarify the situation the ENB (1989: 17) issued a further definition of a mentor as 'a person who would be selected by the student to assist, befriend, guide, advise and counsel' and it was noticeable that the assessment and supervision aspects of the role were not referred to in later documents (ENB 1994). Despite this professional body guidance, mentors were expected to continue to undertake duties as supervisors, assessors and preceptors (Anforth 1992; Andrews 1993; Wilson-Barnett *et al.* 1995), reinforcing the confusion and ambiguities of the role.

What is the current definition of mentorship?

The Nursing and Midwifery Council have addressed the lack of clear definition of preceptorship, supervision and mentorship by releasing a number of explanatory documents (NMC 2002a, 2002b, 2003, 2006, 2008a).

The NMC introduced *Standards to Support Learning and Assessment in Practice* in 2006 (updated in 2008a) for mentors, practice teachers and teachers, which became effective from September 2007, and these have now replaced all previously published standards (NMC 2006, 2008a). There is a single development framework which defines the knowledge and skills to be applied in practice to support and assess students undertaking programmes of study leading to initial registration or a recordable qualification on the professional register.

The current definition of a NMC-recognized **mentor** is:

> a registrant who, following successful completion of an NMC approved mentor preparation programme – or comparable preparation that has been accredited by an Approved Educational Institute (AEI) as meeting the NMC mentor requirements – has achieved the knowledge, skills and competence required to meet the defined outcomes.
>
> (NMC 2008a:19)

Specifically, mentors must demonstrate their knowledge, skills and competence on an ongoing basis to fulfil this important professional role and to remain on the live mentor register.

The standards will be outlined later but it is important to mention that the NMC include assessment as part of a mentor's role. The mentor is accountable for confirming that students have met, or not met, the NMC competencies for continuation on the programme of study or the NMC proficiencies for entry onto the professional nurse register (NMC 2008a). The rest of this chapter will outline what you have to do to meet these standards.

What is the role of the NMC and their requirements for mentors?

The NMC exist to safeguard the health and well-being of the public. This is achieved by:

- ensuring all nurses and midwifes are proficient to work;
- the maintenance of a live professional register;
- setting standards for education, training and ongoing professional development;
- producing a Code of Conduct on how nurses and midwives should perform in their professional role and processes for investigating those who do not.

The requirements for mentors and mentorship are articulated in the Nursing and Midwifery Council (NMC) *Standards to Support Learning and Assessment in Practice* document (NMC 2008a) and should be referred to as the main source for all practitioners. The above elements emerge in these standards as they identify the preparation requirements to become a mentor, the role activities of a mentor and how ongoing competence/development is a necessity in fulfilling this important professional role. For the purpose of this book a summary of the key requirements for mentors will be outlined. These are as follows:

1 Preparation in becoming a mentor
2 Role requirements and responsibilities
3 The role of the sign-off mentor
4 Maintenance of ongoing competence as a mentor

How do you prepare to become a mentor?

All mentors are required to undertake an approved mentor preparation programme. In the past preparatory programmes such as Teaching and Assessing in Clinical Practice (Number 998) would have been approved by local professional bodies such as the English National Board on behalf of the defunct United Kingdom Central Council (replaced by the NMC). However, since 2006 there has been a single developmental **framework to support learning and assessment in practice** (NMC 2008a). Preparatory programmes must encompass these standards, or if a practitioner has undertaken a comparable programme this must have been accredited by an institution of higher education and meet the defined outcomes of the NMC standards.

The developmental framework is 'significant' as it provides a description of the knowledge and skills that are needed to be applied in practice when supporting, teaching and assessing students on NMC programmes. However, it has a second important function for qualified mentors: **The framework can act as a tool to facilitate an ongoing assessment and future development plan to mentors who must maintain and enhance their ongoing competence in fulfilling this important professional role. It is this latter point which underpins the focus and purpose of this book.**

The developmental framework has eight domains which are broad role functions. Each role function is then broken down into specific identified outcomes. For you as a qualified mentor, these domains and outcomes can provide the framework for assessing, developing and demonstrating your ongoing competence and takes account of the NHS *Knowledge and Skills Framework* (DH 2004) upon which many practitioners' job roles are designed. The domains and outcomes are as follows:

Domain 1: Establishing Effective Working Relationships

Outcomes

- Demonstrate an understanding of factors that influence how students integrate into practice settings.
- Provide ongoing and constructive support to facilitate transition from one learning environment to another.
- Have effective professional and inter-professional working relationships to support learning for entry to the register.

Domain 2: Facilitation of Learning

Outcomes

- Use knowledge of the student's stage of learning to select appropriate learning opportunities to meet individual needs.
- Facilitate the selection of appropriate learning strategies to integrate learning from practice and academic experiences.
- Support students in critically reflecting upon their learning experiences in order to enhance future learning.

Domain 3: Assessment and Accountability

Outcomes

- Foster professional growth, personal development and accountability through support of students in practice.
- Demonstrate a breadth of understanding of assessment strategies and the ability to contribute to the total assessment process as part of the teaching team.
- Provide constructive feedback to students and assist them in identifying future learning needs and actions. Manage failing students so that they may enhance their performance and capabilities for safe and effective practice or be able to understand their failure and the implications of this for their future.
- Be accountable for confirming that students have met, or not met, the NMC competencies in practice. As a sign-off mentor confirm that students have met, or not met, the NMC standards of proficiency in practice and are capable of safe and effective practice.

Domain 4: Evaluation of Learning

Outcomes

- Contribute to evaluation of student learning and assessment experiences – proposing aspects for change resulting from such evaluation.
- Participate in **self-evaluation** and **peer evaluation** to facilitate personal development, and contribute to the development of others.

Domain 5: Creating an Environment for Learning

Outcomes

- Support students to identify both learning needs and experiences that are appropriate to their level of learning.
- Use a range of learning experiences, involving patients, clients, carers and the professional team, to meet defined learning needs.

- Identify aspects of the learning environment which could be enhanced – negotiating with others to make appropriate changes.
- Act as a resource to facilitate personal and professional development of others.

Domain 6: Context of Practice

Outcomes

- Contribute to the development of an environment in which effective practice is fostered, implemented, evaluated and disseminated.
- Set and maintain professional boundaries that are sufficiently flexible for providing inter-professional care.
- Initiate and respond to practice developments to ensure safe and effective care is achieved and an effective learning environment is maintained.

Domain 7: Evidence-based Practice

Outcomes

- Identify and apply research and **evidence-based practice** to their area of practice.
- Contribute to strategies to increase or review the evidence base used to support practice.
- Support students in applying an evidence base to their own practice.

Domain 8: Leadership

Outcomes

- Plan a series of learning experiences that will meet students' defined learning needs.
- Be an advocate for students to support them in accessing learning opportunities that meet their individual needs involving a range of other professionals, patients, clients and carers.
- Prioritize work to accommodate support of students within their practice roles.
- Provide **feedback** about the effectiveness of learning and assessment in practice.

(NMC 2008a: Section 2.1.2: 20–21)

What are the role requirements and responsibilities?

As a nurse mentor you must be in the same part or sub-part of the register as the student whom you are teaching, supporting and assessing. This will help to maintain standards in the specific part of the register and ensure students are supported by mentors working and practising at this professional level. You must also practise in the field to which the student is seeking entry, such as adult, child, mental health or learning disability. In the past you may have had personal experience of being supported and assessed by others from a different specialism, which could have resulted in a fragmented learning and assessment experience. The NMC in pursuit of maintaining professional standards and public protection are keen to prevent this in the future so that students seeking registration or a recordable qualification are taught and assessed as proficient by mentors working in the same specialist field of practice. Further guidance on this can be located in the NMC Circular 26/2007, accessible from the NMC website at http://www.nmc-uk.org/.

You will find that numerous sources can provide this information such as:

- discussions with other mentors;
- discussions with the local university;
- reviewing other documents such as the Royal College of Nursing *Guidance for Mentors of Nursing Students and Midwives* (RCN 2007) and the NMC *Standards to Support Learning and Assessment in Practice* (NMC 2008a).

Some key responsibilities may include the need to:

- familiarize yourself with the student's programme of study, the stage of their training/education, the student's record of achievement to date and the practice assessment documentation;
- identify, select, support and assess a range of learning opportunities in the placement area which are congruent with what the student has to achieve;
- organize, co-ordinate and observe students' learning activities and nursing practical skills (note that a minimum 40 per cent of a student's time on placement must be spent being supervised (directly or indirectly) by a mentor);
- supervise students in learning situations, provide constructive feedback and suggest how improvements could be made;
- communicate with others (such as mentors, practice facilitators, practice teachers or personal tutors) who have a vested interest in a student's performance and record this accordingly;
- analyse evidence from a variety of sources for making judgements about the competence/proficiency of students (including knowledge, skills and attitudes) and be accountable for such decisions;
- record all meetings, discussions, progress and untoward incidents or concerns about students' achievements and provide evidence as required of this;
- maintain your ongoing competence as a mentor and ensure these details are maintained on the local mentor register (the register is now held by the practice placement provider, not the higher education institution).

This list can be endless! An effective way for you as a mentor to continue assessing and judging, if you are meeting your professional responsibilities, is by using the NMC domains and learning outcomes from the NMC standards (2008a) outlined earlier as a framework to guide you.

What is the role of the sign-off mentor?

The NMC (2008a) require the final assessment of a student's performance to gain entry to the register or achieve a recordable qualification to be completed by mentors who are designated as **sign-off mentors**. If you are a qualified mentor but not a sign-off mentor you can assess students on programmes of study up to the final placement; the final assessment of practice can involve your input but *must* be completed by those who are registered as a sign-off mentor. Sign-off mentors must be on the same part or sub-part of the register that the student is intending to join.

If you wish to become a sign-off mentor the NMC have identified criteria for the role (NMC standards 2008a: Section 2.1.3). These criteria incorporate the role requirements/responsibilities outlined above with the addition that mentors have:

- clinical currency and capability in the field of practice;
- been supervised on at least three occasions for signing off proficiency by a recognized sign-off mentor;
- an in-depth knowledge of their accountability to the NMC when making decisions about students' proficiency levels at the end of their programme for entry to the register or a recordable qualification;
- their details as a sign-off mentor recorded on the local mentor register.

How do you maintain your ongoing competence as a mentor?

The NMC are very specific in the regulatory standards set out for mentors to demonstrate their own ongoing competence. There are two **mandatory** elements to this:

Annual updating

After qualifying as a mentor you must maintain your knowledge, skills and competence through regular updating (which is in fact annual updating) in relation to these outcomes (NMC 2008a: Section 3.2.2). The NMC (2008a: 30) indicate that the purpose of annual updating is to ensure mentors:

a) Have current knowledge of NMC approved programmes
b) Are able to discuss the implications of changes to NMC programmes
c) Have an opportunity to discuss issues relating to mentoring, assessment of competence and fitness for safe and effective practice.

There are many ways you can update annually, which we will explore later in the book. For instance, we provide case studies for you to analyse and use for updating. They can be analysed in relation to the eight NMC domains and outcomes for mentors (NMC 2008a). Further on in the book there are more activities and sources of evidence that you can use for your own updates and to demonstrate your ongoing competence.

Triennial review

The NMC (2008a) have indicated that every mentor will be subject to a triennial review which may be part of an employer-led appraisal system if they wish (or are required by their employer as part of their job role) to remain on the local register.

At this triennial review, each mentor must have evidence of having:

- Mentored at least two students with due regard (extenuating circumstances permitting) within a three-year period.
- Participated in annual updating – to include an opportunity to meet and explore assessment and supervision issues with other mentors/ practice teachers.
- Explored as a group activity the validity and reliability of judgements made when assessing practice in challenging circumstances.
- Mapped ongoing development in their role against the current NMC mentor standards.
- Been deemed to have met all requirements needed to be maintained on the local register as a mentor or sign-off mentor.

(NMC 2008a:12)

Why is there a need for mentors to maintain their ongoing competence?

Several factors have arguably contributed to the introduction of this requirement. First, Duffy completed a study in 2003 which identified that mentors were 'failing to fail' students. Several reasons were presented including giving students the benefit of the doubt as they were at an early stage in their training and might resolve their problems as they continued in the programme; at the other end of the continuum some mentors indicated that they did not want to be responsible for ending a student's career if they were at the end of their course, and consequently passed their assessment. The fear of the university's appeal system was also expressed in the study as mentors felt 'pressurized' into passing a student, which may have been at odds with their professional judgement (Duffy 2003). The implications of such actions raise concerns about public protection as incompetent practitioners may enter the professional register; there is also a clear breach by mentors of the Code of Professional Conduct (NMC 2008b).

Secondly, concerns were also being expressed by employers about registrants'

fitness for practice (UKCC 1994, 1999; Hewison and Wildman 1996). There were overlapping issues around the quality and nature of the support students were receiving in practice and the judgements being made about students' fitness within practice to gain entry to the professional register. The NMC therefore decided to set up two projects on a new standard to support learning and assessment in practice (NMC 2004) and fitness for practice (NMC 2005) at the point of registration. Both reports produced significant changes to the activities required from mentors in assessing student competence and maintaining their own level of competence in order to remain on the professional register.

Thirdly, mentors have been required by the NMC to attend an educational update despite the lack of guidance on the content and nature of this updating activity. Pressures of work are often cited as a reason for poor attendance at these events but of greater significance is the lack of evidence that mentors' practices change following attendance at an educational update event (Nolan *et al.* 2000).

What happens if a mentor does not update?

In the future this will no longer be acceptable as mentors will need to produce evidence of updating activities if they wish to remain on the local live mentor register and fulfil both their professional and contractual employment responsibilities. If mentors do not update and are removed from the live register it is conceivable that this could have implications for meeting the NHS Knowledge and Skills Gateways (DH 2003, 2004), their job descriptions and their role as an employee of the Trust.

Whilst NMC quality assurances processes have not analysed how mentor updating activities contribute to the ongoing development and practices of mentors in supporting students, this issue lies at the core of ongoing competence development (Bradshaw 1998; Andre 2000) and, potentially, of continuing employment as a nurse.

Summary

The aim of this chapter has been to provide a review of mentorship within a United Kingdom context.

Key points

- The history of mentorship reveals some difficulties within the UK on defining it as a concept and outlining its role functions.
- The requirements for mentors and mentorship are now articulated in the Nursing and Midwifery Council (NMC) *Standards to Support Learning and Assessment in Practice* document (NMC 2008a).
- The standards are written in the format of a developmental framework which provides a description of the knowledge and skills that are needed to

be applied in practice when supporting, teaching and assessing students on NMC programmes.

- The developmental framework can also act as a tool to facilitate an ongoing assessment and future development plan to mentors who must maintain and enhance their ongoing competence in fulfilling this important professional role.
- Mentors will have to demonstrate to the employers through a triennial review how they have maintained their ongoing competence through annual updating activities to remain on the live mentor register.
- Mentors who do not update will be removed from the live register and this may have implications for promotion and their ability to meet the requirements of their job role.
- Mentors must be in the same part or sub-part of the register as the student and also be practising in the field to which the student is seeking entry, such as adult, child, mental health or learning disability nursing.
- The NMC (2008a) require the final assessment of a student's performance to gain entry to the register or achieve a recordable qualification to be completed by mentors who are designated as **sign-off mentors**.

The following chapter will explore in more detail the concept of competence that is essential to performance. It will explore the measurement of competence and the civil 'standard of proof' used by the NMC when judgements about competence and fitness to practise occur. The chapter will also outline how ongoing competence as a mentor could be linked to an employer-led appraisal system incorporating the National Health Service (NHS) Knowledge and Skills Framework (DH 2004).

References

Andre, K. (2000) Grading student clinical performance: the Australian perspective, *Nurse Education Today*, 20: 672–9.

Andrews, M. (1993) A qualitative study exploring the relationship between support, supervision and clinical learning for Project 2000 students. Unpublished MSc dissertation, University of Manchester.

Andrews, M. (1999) Mentorship in nursing: a literature review, *Journal of Advanced Nursing*, 29(1): 201–7.

Anforth, P. (1992) Mentors not assessors, *Nurse Education Today*, 12: 299–302.

Armitage, P. and Burnard, P. (1991) Mentors or preceptors? Narrowing the theory–practice gap, *Nurse Education Today*, 11(3): 225–9.

Barlow, S. (1991) Impossible dream, *Nursing Times*, 87(1): 53–4.

Bracken, E. and Davis, J. (1989) The implications of mentorship in nursing career development, *Senior Nurse*, 9: 15–16.

Bradshaw, A. (1998) Defining 'competency' in nursing (part II): an analytical review, *Journal of Clinical Nursing*, 7(2): 103–11.

Clutterbuck, D. (1985) *Everybody Seeks a Mentor: How to Foster Talent Within the Organisation.* London: Institute of Personnel Management.

DH (Department of Health) (2003) *Agenda for Change.* London: Department of Health.

DH (2004) *The NHS Knowledge and Skills Framework and Development Review Process.* London: Department of Health.

Donovan, J. (1990) The concept and role of mentor, *Nurse Education Today*, 10 (4): 274–9.

Duffy, K. (2003) *Failing Students: A Qualitative Study of Factors that Influence the Decisions Regarding Assessment of Students' Competence in Practice.* London: NMC.

ENB (English National Board for Nursing Midwifery and Health Visiting) (1987) *Institutional and Course Approval/Reapproval Process. Information Required, Criteria and Guidelines.* Circular 1987/28/MAT. London: English National Board for Nursing Midwifery and Health Visiting.

ENB (1988) *Institutional and Course Approval/Reapproval Process. Information Required, Criteria and Guidelines.* Circular 1988/39/APS. London: English National Board for Nursing Midwifery and Health Visiting.

ENB (1989) *Preparation of Teachers, Practitioner Teachers, Mentors and Supervisors in the Context of Project 2000.* London: English National Board for Nursing Midwifery and Health Visiting.

ENB (1994) *News Issue*, 14. London: English National Board for Nursing Midwifery and Health Visiting.

Foy, H. and Waltho, B. (1989) The mentor system: are learner nurses benefiting?, *Senior Nurse*, 9 (5): 24–5.

Hewison, A. and Wildman, S. (1996) The theory practice gap in nursing: a new dimension, *Journal of Advanced Nursing*, 24 (4): 754–61.

Jinks, A.M. and Williams, R.H. (1994) Evaluation of a community staff preparation strategy for the teaching assessing and mentorship of Project 2000 diploma students, *Nurse Education Today*, 14: 44–51.

Maggs, C. (1994) Mentorship in nursing and midwifery education: issues for research, *Nurse Education Today*, 14: 22–9.

Melia, K. (1987) *Working and Learning.* London: Tavistock.

Morle, K. (1990) Mentorship: is it the case of the emperor's new clothes or a rose by any other name?, *Nurse Education Today*, 10: 66–9.

Morris, N., John, G. and Keen, T. (1988) Mentors: learning the ropes, *Nursing Times*, 64 (46): 24–6.

Myrick, F. (1988) Preceptorship: is it the answer to problems in clinical teaching?, *Journal of Advanced Nursing*, 13: 588–91.

Neary, M., Phillips, R. and Davies, B. (1994) *The Practitioner Teacher: A Study in the Introduction of Mentors in the Pre-registration Nurse Education Programme in Wales.* Cardiff: School of Education, University of Wales.

NMC (Nursing and Midwifery Council) (2002a) *Supporting Nurses and Midwives through Lifelong Learning.* London: NMC.

NMC (2002b) *Standards for the Preparation of Teachers of Nursing and Midwifery.* London: NMC.

NMC (2003) *Preceptorship.* London: NMC.

NMC (2004) *Consultation on a Standard to Support Learning and Assessment in Practice.* London: NMC.

NMC (2005) *Consultation on Fitness for Practice at the Point of Registration.* London: NMC.

NMC (2006) *Standards to Support Learning and Assessment in Practice*. London: NMC.

NMC (2007) *Applying Due Regard to Learning and Assessment in Practice*. NMC Circular 26/ 2007. http://www.nmc-uk.org/ (Accessed 24 September 2009) London: NMC.

NMC (2008a) *Standards to Support Learning and Assessment in Practice*. http://www.nmc-uk.org/aDisplayDocument.aspx?documentID=4368 (Accessed 10 July 2009) London: NMC.

NMC (2008b) *The Code: Standards of Conduct, Performance and Ethics for Nurses and Midwives*. http://www.nmc-uk.org/aArticle.aspx?ArticleID=3056 (Accessed 10 July 2009). London: NMC.

Nolan, M., Owen, R., Curran, M. and Venables, A. (2000) Reconceptualising the outcomes of Continuing Professional Development, *International Journal of Nursing Studies*, 37: 457–67.

RCN (Royal College of Nursing) (2007) *Guidance for Mentors of Nursing Students and Midwives*. London: RCN.

Shamian, J. and Inhaber, R. (1985) The concept and practice of preceptorship in contemporary nursing: a review of pertinent literature, *International Journal of Nursing Studies*, 22 (2): 79–88.

Shamian, J. and Lemieux, S. (1984) An evaluation of the preceptorship model versus the formal teaching model, *The Journal of Continuing Education in Nursing*, 15 (3): 86–9.

UKCC (United Kingdom Central Council for Nursing, Midwifery and Health Visiting) (1994) *The Future of Professional Practice: The Council's Standards for Education and Practice following Registration*. London: UKCC.

UKCC (1999) *Fitness for Practice*. London: UKCC.

Wilson-Barnett, J., Butterworth, T., White, E., Twinn, S., Davies, S. and Riley, L. (1995) Clinical support and the Project 2000 nursing student: factors influencing this process, *Journal of Advanced Nursing*, 21: 1152–8.

WNB (Welsh National Board for Nursing, Midwifery and Health Visiting) (1992) *Mentors, Preceptors and Supervisors: Their Place in Nursing, Midwifery and Health Visiting*. Cardiff: WNB.

2

The Nature of Competence

Karen Staniland and Cyril Murray

Aim

The aim of this chapter is to explore the concept of competence and the relationship between ongoing competence, mentor updating and employer-led appraisals.

Learning outcomes

After reading this chapter you will be able to:

- identify the concepts associated with 'competence' and its measurement;
- discuss the legal definition of competence and the NMC Standard of Proof;
- identify the background context as to why competence as a mentor could be linked to an emloyer-led appraisal.

What is competence?

The *Encarta English Dictionary* (2009) defines competence as 'the ability to do something well, measured against a standard, especially ability acquired through experience or training.' This gives a broad understanding of the word *but* you will find that the literature also offers many ambiguous and confusing definitions of competence and that there is no nationally *accepted* description and little consensus on the subject (Ashworth and Morrison 1991; While 1994; Eraut and du Boulay 1999; Dunn *et al.* 2000; Cowan *et al.* 2005; Defloor *et al.* 2006; King's College London 2009). McMullan *et al.* (2003) and Cowan *et al.* (2005) also state that associated terms such as competency, capability and performance are used inconsistently and often interchangeably. It is interesting therefore to review various concepts of competence in this chapter in order to understand some of the difficulties that might be experienced with its measurement.

Some definitions of competence are based upon a description of an action or an outcome of performance (McMullan *et al.* 2003) in which the ability to perform a task incorporates both capability and performance (Redfern *et al.* 2002). A relevant example of this can be taken from the work of Patricia Benner (1984), who defined *nursing* competency as the ability to perform a task with desirable outcomes under the varied circumstances of the real world. A 'competent' level in this context identifies a step in the process of acquiring a higher level of proficiency. Competent practitioners in her view are consciously able to plan their actions, but lack flexibility and speed (Benner 1984). Conceptually, competence here assumes the integration of knowledge skills and attitudes within clinical practice (Meretoja *et al.* 2004; Defloor *et al.* 2006) and this is associated with the *direct* observation of a performance (King's College London 2009).

However, this approach has been criticized as being fragmented and **reductionist** (simplified), focusing upon what individuals can do at the expense of the links between tasks and the performance in practice (Gonczi 1994; Scholes *et al.* 2000). Cassidy (2009) illustrates this by using an example of the administration of an injection. The behavioural skill of administering an injection follows safe policy and procedure but the invasive activity can impact upon a patient's anxiety, privacy and dignity, which necessitate the implementation of other attributes including problem solving and critical thinking abilities in demonstrating competence.

It is suggested by some (Le Var 1996 and Eraut 1994, 1998) that clinical practice cannot be measured by using a behavioural or outcome approach. Le Var and Eraut have indicated that 'performance' is concerned with the ability to do 'something' but it is unclear if this demonstrates competence and whether competence indicates a greater degree of ability than capability or vice versa.

Another perspective on defining competence is based upon a generic approach associated with a cluster of attributes and abilities (critical thinking, problem solving, transferability etc.) that are essential to performance (Watson *et al.* 2002; Dolan 2003; Defloor *et al.* 2006). Cassidy (2009: 41) indicates that 'an attribute approach to assessing competence therefore might place as much value on the way a student assists an incapacitated person to eat, as it does on his or her knowledge of nutrition'. Criticisms of this approach include concerns about the existence of such attributes, their transferability and whether concepts such as critical thinking can be measured to determine competence

(Gonczi 1994; Norman *et al.* 2002; Watson *et al.* 2002; Clinton *et al.* 2005; Cassidy 2009).

If these definitions of competence are considered confusing, it is important to also consider the legal implications in the measurement of competence.

What is the legal definition of competence?

The **Bolam test** is a familiar concept in medical practice as a measure of whether the doctor has discharged his or her standard of care in the management of the patient, but it is important to realize that it also applies to all professionals, not just doctors. In the English law of tort (tort law is the name that is given to a body of law that creates and provides remedies for civil wrongs that do not arise out of contractual duties) the Bolam test is one of the rules used to determine the issue of professional negligence.

This test came into being through a series of English cases culminating in *Bolam v Friern Hospital Management Committee* (1957) 1 WLR 582 (Shanmugam 2002: 007). It has since also been advanced and explained further in subsequent cases. This test will judge whether a practitioner falls below the appropriate standard of what a reasonable person would do in those circumstances, although he/she is not measured by the best:

> The burden is discharged by calling expert evidence to show what other professionals, of similar standing and exercising that particular skill, would have done in that situation.
>
> (Shanmugam 2002: 7)

Take, for example, a situation where a mentor who had undertaken a mentor course would have been deemed competent to assess student nurses. During an assessment of a student nurse there was clear evidence that the student was not competent in a specific skill, such as moving and handling a patient into and out of a bath. However, the mentor decided to give the student the benefit of the doubt as the student was early on in her training and had time to improve. In the next placement the new mentor looked at the student passport and, in discussion with the student, identified those skills she was deemed to be competent in. The student was delegated some work activities in relation to patient care by the new mentor which included moving and handling patients into and out of a bath. An accident occurred in which a patient slipped out of the hoist, banged his head and later died from his injury as the equipment had not been properly used. The patient's relatives later sued the hospital and upon subsequent investigation it came to light that the student had not been assessed by either of the mentors as being competent in this nursing skill. Both nurses would have been subject to the Bolam test here if professional negligence was deemed to have occurred and it is likely they would be disciplined internally and reported to the NMC.

The NMC Standard of Proof

Within the United Kingdom, guidance from the professional bodies on the subject of competence had been vague (Bradshaw 1997) in that incompetence is viewed as 'a lack of knowledge, skill or judgement of such a nature that a registrant is unfit to practise safely and effectively in any field in which they claim to be qualified to practise or seek to practise' (NMC 2004: 3) and competence is regarded as performing 'behaviour' safely and effectively. For instance, it is stated that, to practise competently, 'You must possess the knowledge, skills and abilities required for lawful, safe and effective practice without direct supervision' (NMC 2008a: 4) However, the NMC introduced a 'Standard of Proof' amendment (NMC 2008b) which would be used in situations of competence, as will now be explained.

The Department of Health (DH 2007a) published a White Paper *Trust, Assurance and Safety – The Regulation of Health Professionals in the Twenty-first Century* in February 2007. This paper clarified the government's plan for modernizing professional regulation, to ensure continuing confidence in healthcare professionals.

Some relevant developments from the White Paper are in the Health and Social Care Bill (DH 2007b) which came into effect on 3 November 2008. One of these developments was the introduction of the civil standard of proof for Fitness to Practise hearings for all health and social care regulators. Before this date, NMC Fitness to Practise hearings utilized the criminal 'standard of proof': this required the facts of any allegation to be proved 'beyond all reasonable doubt', in that however serious the allegation, the same standard of proof was required. However, a NMC Fitness to Practise hearing is not a criminal court; it is a professional regulatory hearing and the criminal standard is not appropriate in these circumstances. The *civil* standard of proof is based 'on the balance of probabilities' – but the whole idea of this standard is that it must be flexibly applied. The evidence submitted might change in this context and the consequences are more serious if the allegation is proved (NMC 2008b).

What does this mean for me?

Mentors will have been deemed competent under the NMC standards (2008c) by having undergone extra training. Mentors therefore would be expected to follow the regulations governing the progress of students and have a responsibility to their higher education institutions by upholding these set regulations. Potentially a mentor could be challenged on the grounds that a student assessment was unfair. This then would be measured by the principles of the standard of proof if there was a dispute on what standards were followed in the assessment.

However, it is important to consider that this could also work in the opposite way. A lazy mentor, who passes a student because it is too much trouble to refer them, could be viewed as acting negligently. Failing to take care in the giving of information when knowledge is relied on by a recipient who subsequently suffers harm (as in a student who is not safe but deemed safe by a lazy mentor and who would put patients and others at risk) is professionally unacceptable (NMC 2008a).

So whilst it can be identified that the concepts of competence and competencies within nursing are wide open to interpretation, defining how they may be measured appears to be just as challenging. This is identified in work by Harden *et al.* (1975), Andre (2000), Stronach *et al.* (2002) and Watson *et al.* (2002).

So, how do we measure student competence?

Stronach *et al.* (2002) state that the measurement of competence by the appraiser is difficult and, even if reliable and valid tools were developed, Watson *et al.* (2002: 423) suggest that 'the issue of what level of performance indicates competence and at what level a student can be deemed incompetent remains unresolved'. You have probably identified already that observation is often used as an assessment tool for student competence.

Observation

Sims (1976) reported that it is possible to make inferences about an individual's general competence on the basis of an observed performance in a limited number of situations but the validity of this statement is questioned by While (1994). The Australian Nursing Council Incorporated (ANCI) (University of Queensland Department of Education 1990), as reported by Dunn *et al.* (2000), regards competency as an intangible construct which cannot be directly observed. This would be consistent with the earlier perspectives which define competence based upon a cluster of attributes and abilities.

Gonczi *et al.* (1993) agree that competence cannot be observed directly but added to the debate by proposing that it is 'inferred' from 'performance'. Hence, under a performance-based assessment system, as in an assessment of student nurses, assessors will judge, from evidence based on performance, specifically whether an individual meets criteria specified in competence standards (in this context these might be viewed as the student's assessment documentation). However, it remains questionable as to the applicability of such a requirement in what is increasingly a very turbulent practice environment. Mentors reading this book are probably very familiar with the time pressures and constraints which are often perceived to be barriers to such activities taking place (Rutherford et al. 2005).

Bearing these opinions in mind, it is useful also to remember that most assessments of student competence in practice should be undertaken through direct observation by mentors (NMC 2008c). It is important to keep in mind as well that direct observation can also be useful in mapping performance against the desired competency level for that role/function/level in order to identify any gaps in the student's knowledge, skill or attitude and this also gives the mentor an opportunity to intervene appropriately. This can then decrease the 'openness' of the interpretation of an observation and identify a student's learning needs.

So far we have talked about the difficulties for a mentor in assessing a student's competence due to the varied definitions of what competence actually is. In the next section we turn to recent initiatives in the ongoing measurement of a *mentor's* competence which can be linked to an employer's appraisal in order for them to stay on the live register.

How do we measure a mentor's competence?

It is evident that healthcare organizations are continually reorganizing their services in which line management structures may include non-nursing personnel performing reviews about job roles and performance of nursing staff. Literature on measuring the clinical competence of nurses within Australia (Dunn et al. 2000) and Belgium (Defloor et al. 2006) indicates the need for reliable and valid assessments reflecting the reality of the clinical context and incorporating the problem-solving processes used by the clinician.

Interestingly, it could be argued that when applied to the measurement of *mentors'* abilities within the clinical learning environment context, these non-nursing appraisers would possess limited professional insight into the role and would be challenged to make judgements about the knowledge, skills and abilities of mentors for effective practice in supporting student nurses.

General updating, mentor competence and the reviewer perspective

In order to develop the activities of maintaining mentor competence it is first necessary to explain some of the background for general updating, mentor competence and the reviewer perspective. This is introduced here and the way it might be implemented is explained in more detail in Chapter 3.

Agenda for Change

The government introduced *Agenda for Change* in 2003 (DH 2003). The government's intention here was that every nurse would link their own professional development with competencies and annual performance development reviews. These appraisal reviews grade the individual, their performance and the role itself (DH 2004; Berridge *et al.* 2007) and have close links to pay and career enhancement.

The Knowledge and Skills Framework

Agenda for Change (DH 2003) produced a key tool – The National Health Service (NHS) Knowledge and Skills Framework (KSF) (DH 2004). This framework provided a range of competencies which can be specifically designed to each practitioner's role and focused upon the application of the knowledge and skills to meet the demands of their job role. If you are a qualified mentor, mentoring students is considered part of your job role. The NHS KSF 'has been designed to form the basis of a developmental review process' which is 'an ongoing cycle of review, planning, development and evaluation of all staff in the NHS' (DH 2004: 13). The developmental review process should link with the current employers' appraisal system so that '*the two work seamlessly together to support an individual's development*' (DH 2004: 14).

The NMC (2008c) requires every mentor to undertake a **triennial review** which may be part of an employer-led appraisal system if they wish (or as part of their job role) in order to remain on the **local register**. The developmental framework (Stage 2 of the NMC 2008c Standards) describes the knowledge and skills practitioners need to apply when they facilitate, teach and assess students in practice (NMC 2008c). Mentors will have to demonstrate to their employers through an appraisal scheme how they have updated their knowledge, skills and competence if they wish to remain on the local mentor register. Specific examples of how this might be done are detailed in the following chapter.

It would appear logical, then, that any development review also includes a review about the ongoing competence of a mentor as identified in the following section.

Employer appraisal systems

By linking the triennial review to an NHS KSF review, the evidence presented by a mentor could potentially ascertain whether updating activities have led to changes to the performance of that mentor and how they have applied their knowledge, skills and competence within their job role. It could also provide the individual with an opportunity to evaluate their own practice and act as a motivator for future development.

We have already mentioned that employers now have a responsibility to ensure that staff have the necessary knowledge, skills and competence within their job role and to support their development needs as necessary. Any judgement made about a mentor's performance as part of an appraisal must be transparent, addressing concern where appropriate and ultimately be utilized for adding and removing individuals from the local register, as will be explained in Chapter 3.

It is worth mentioning that, to date, implementation of these reforms from *Agenda for Change* (DH 2003) have been patchy nationally, with over half of all nurses missing out on a career development scheme (Snow 2009). The National Audit Watchdog found that 46 per cent of nurses in 2008 had not received a knowledge and skills review (Snow 2009) and recommended that all nurses should be requesting, even demanding, one.

Summary

The aim of this chapter was to explore the concept of competence and the relationship between ongoing competence, mentor updating and employer-led appraisals.

Key points

- There are many difficulties in the interpretation of the word competence and legal and professional issues need to be considered.
- Employers now have a responsibility to ensure that staff apply the necessary knowledge, skills and competence within their job role and to support their developmental needs as necessary.

- Measurement of the competence of a mentor might be combined with an employer's appraisal scheme in the form of a triennial review in order for a mentor to remain on the live register.

The following chapter will concentrate more on the *detail* of an employer's appraisal scheme and give some practical examples of how reviewers can make judgements with regard to a mentor's competence.

References

Andre, K. (2000) Grading student clinical performance: the Australian perspective, *Nurse Education Today*, 20: 672–9.

Ashworth, P. and Morrison, P. (1991) Problems of competence-based nurse education, *Nurse Education Today*, 11(4): 256–60.

Benner, P. (1984) *From Novice To Expert: Excellence and Power in Clinical Nursing Practice.* Menlo Park, CA: Addison Wesley.

Berridge, E.J., Kelly, D. and Gould, D. (2007) Staff appraisal and continuing professional development, *Journal of Research in Nursing*, 12 (1): 57–70.

Bradshaw, A. (1997) Defining competency in nursing (Part 1): a policy review, *Journal of Clinical Nursing*, 6: 347–54.

Cassidy, S. (2009) Interpretation of competence in student assessment, *Nursing Standard*, 23 (18): 39–46.

Clinton, M., Murrells, T. and Robinson, S. (2005) Assessing competence in nursing: a comparison of nurses prepared through degree and diploma programmes, *Journal of Clinical Nursing*, 14 (1): 82–94.

Cowan, D.T., Norman, I. and Coopamah, V.P. (2005) Competence in nursing practice: a controversial concept – a focused review of literature, *Nurse Education Today*, 25 (5): 355–62.

Defloor, T., Van Hecke, A., Verhaeghe, S., Gobert, M., Darras, E. and Grypdonck, M. (2006) The clinical nursing competences and their complexity in Belgian general hospitals, *Journal of Advanced Nursing*, 56 (6): 669–78.

DH (Department of Health) (2003) *Agenda For Change.* London: Department of Health.

DH (2004) *The NHS Knowledge and Skills Framework and Development Review Process.* London: Department of Health.

DH (2007a) *Trust, Assurance and Safety – The Regulation of Health Professionals in the 21st Century.* http://www.dh.gov.uk/en/Publicationsandstatistics/Publications/PublicationsPolicyAndGuidance/DH_065946 (Accessed 10 July 2009).

DH (2007b) *The Health and Social Care Act.* http://www.dh.gov.uk/en/Publicationsandstatistics/Legislation/Actsandbills/HealthandSocialCareBill/index.htm (Accessed 10 July 2009).

Dolan, G. (2003) Assessing student competency: will we ever get it right?, *Journal of Clinical Nursing*, 12: 132–41.

Dunn, S.V., Lawson, D., Robertson, S., Underwood, M., Clark, R. Valentine, T. *et al.*

(2000) The development of competency standards for specialist critical care nurses, *Journal of Advanced Nursing*, 31 (2): 339–46.

Encarta English Dictionary (2009). http://www.encarta.msn.co.uk/encnet/features/dictionary/DictionaryResults.aspx?lextype=3&search=competence (Accessed 24 November 2009).

Eraut, M. (1994) *Developing Professional Knowledge and Competence*. London: Falmer Press.

Eraut, M. (1998) Concepts of competence, *Journal of Interprofessional Care*, 12: 127–39.

Eraut, M. and du Bolay, B. (1999) *Developing the Attributes of Medical Professional Judgement and Competence*. London: Department of Health.

Gonczi, A., Hager, P. and Athanasou, J. (1993) *A Guide to the Development of Competency-based Assessment Strategies for the Professions*, Research Paper 8. Canberra: AGPS.

Gonczi, A. (1994) Competency-based assessments in the professions in Australia, *Assessment in Education*, 1 (1): 27–44.

Harden, R., Stevenson, M., Wilson Downie, W. and Wilson, G. (1975) Assessment of clinical competence using objective structured examination, *British Medical Journal*, 1: 447–51.

King's College London (2009) Nursing competence: what are we assessing and how should it be measured? *Policy Plus Evidence, Issues and Opinions in Healthcare*, 18: June. http://www.klc.ac.uk/schools/nursing/nnru/policy (Accessed 6 July 2009).

Le Var, R.M. (1996) NVQs in nursing, midwifery and health visiting: a question of assessment and learning, *Nurse Education Today*, 16: 85–93.

McMullan, M., Endacott, R., Gray, M., Jasper, M., Miller, C.l., Scholes, J. *et al.* (2003) Portfolios and assessment of competence: a review of the literature, *Journal of Advanced Nursing*, 41 (3): 283–94.

Meretoja, R., Isoaho, H. and Leino-Kilpi, H. (2004) Nurse competence scale: development and psychometric testing, *Journal of Advanced Nursing*, 47: 124–33.

NMC (Nursing and Midwifery Council) (2004) *Reporting Lack of Competence: A Guide for Employers and Managers*. London: NMC.

NMC (2008a) *The Code: Standards of Conduct, Performance and Ethics for Nurses and Midwives*. http://www.nmc-uk.org/aArticle.aspx?ArticleID=3056 (Accessed 10 July 2009).

NMC (2008b) *Using the Civil Standard of Proof*. http://www.nmc-uk.org/aArticle.aspx?ArticleID=3141 (Accessed 10 July 2009).

NMC (2008c) *Standards to Support Learning and Assessment in Practice, NMC Standards for Mentors, Practice Teachers and Teachers*. http://www.nmc-uk.org/aDisplayDocument.aspx?documentID=4368 (Accessed 10 July 2009).

Norman, I.J., Watson, R., Murrells, T., Calman, L. and Redfern, S. (2002) The validity and reliability of methods to assess the competence to practise of pre-registration nursing and midwifery students, *International Journal of Nursing*, 39 (2): 133–45.

Redfern, S., Norman, I., Calman, L., Watson, R. and Murrells, T. (2002) Assessing competence to practise in nursing: a review of the literature, *Research Papers in Education*, 17: 51–77.

Rutherford, J., Leigh, J., Monk, J. and Murray, C. (2005) Creating an organizational infrastructure to develop and support new nursing roles – a framework for debate, *Journal of Nursing Management*, 13: 97–105.

Scholes, J., Endacott, R. and Chellel, A. (2000) A formula for diversity: a review of critical care curriculum, *Journal of Clinical Nursing*, 9: 382–90.

Shanmugam, K. (2002) Testing the Bolam test: consequences of recent developments,

Singapore Medical Journal, 43(1): 007–011, http://www.sma.org.sg/smj/4301/4301l1.pdf (Accessed 10 July 2009).

Sims, A. (1976) The critical incident technique in evaluating student nurse performance, *International Journal of Nursing Studies*, 13: 123–30.

Snow, T. (2009) Almost half of NHS staff are missing out on career development scheme, *Nursing Standard*, 23 (23): 13–14.

Stronach, I., Corbin, B., McNamara, O., Stark, S. and Warne, T. (2002) Towards an uncertain politics of professionalism: teacher and nurse identities in flux, *Journal of Education Policy*, 17 (2): 109–38.

University of Queensland Department of Education, Assessment and Evaluation Research Unit (1990) *ANRAC Nursing Competencies Assessment Project: Report to the Australasian Nurse Registration Authorities Conferences*. North Adelaide: ANRAC.

Watson, R., Stimpson, A., Topping, A. and Porock, D. (2002) Clinical competence assessment in nursing: a systematic review of the literature, *Journal of Advanced Nursing*, 39(5): 421–31.

While, A. (1994) Competence versus performance: which is more important?, *Journal of Advanced Nursing*, 20: 525–31.

3

Mentorship: Practice Placement Provider Perspectives and Responsibilities

Karen Staniland and Mary Douglas

Aim

This chapter will outline the organizational and reviewer requirements, from the practice placement provider perspective, in addressing the ongoing competence of mentors.

Learning outcomes

After reading this chapter you will be able to:

- outline the organizational and reviewer obligations in promoting and recording the ongoing competence of mentors;
- discuss the role of the reviewer in the review/appraisal process;
- examine the concepts associated with making judgements on:

  ➢ the types of evidence which may be produced by a mentor to demonstrate competence;
  ➢ the quality and robustness of the evidence produced.

Introduction

Any nursing programme combines academic study at the university (education providers) with clinical placements (**practice placement providers**) from a wide variety of service settings, specialisms and locations that mirror the diverse roles and responsibilities in the arena of nursing care. Practice placement providers maintain these clinical placement areas. Universities usually have link lecturer representatives with practice placements and qualified mentors are responsible for the students' learning and supervision whilst they are on placement. We have established in previous chapters that there is a single developmental framework to support learning and assessment in practice which defines and describes the knowledge and skills registrants need to apply in practice when they support and assess students. The NMC (2008) have identified outcomes for mentors, practice teachers and teachers so that there is clear accountability for making decisions that lead to entry to the register. However, these activities cannot be performed without support. The purpose of this chapter is to make the organizational obligations of the practice placement providers clear, to enable mentors to fulfil their role. These obligations are outlined by the NMC (2006, 2008).

In the past, Schools of Nursing within universities have been responsible for maintaining an up-to-date register of current mentors. Since implementation of the NMC standards in 2006, which were updated in 2008, this commitment was passed on to practice placement providers, who now have specific obligations.

This chapter will consider the professional and organizational obligations related to promoting and recording the ongoing competence of mentors. It will then outline the role of a 'reviewer' in the review/appraisal process and will discuss the concepts associated with making judgements on the type, quality and robustness of the evidence produced by mentors.

What are these professional and organizational obligations?

Practice placement providers are required to have relevant systems in place to monitor and update their mentors appropriately. That is, practice placement providers are expected to keep records and be able to produce evidence to NMC visitors during review visits. This evidence needs to demonstrate assurance that the mentors on their register have updated themselves and can fulfil their professional responsibilities to mentor students.

Specifically, practice placement providers are responsible for:

- Holding and maintaining an up-to-date register of current mentors and practice teachers.
- Regularly reviewing the register and adding or removing names of registrants as necessary.
- Ensuring that all mentors who are designated as sign-off mentors are annotated as such on the local register.
- Providing confirmation through the mentor register to the education provider that there are sufficient mentors who meet the NMC standards to adequately support the number of students on placement across the organization.

(NMC 2008)

Education providers should use the (local) register to confirm that there are sufficient mentors and practice teachers who meet the NMC standards to support learning and assessment in practice and the number of students undertaking the range of NMC-approved programmes currently being offered.

The NMC also requires the practice placement provider, in partnership with education providers, to make provision for the annual updating of registrants. This updating can be provided in a variety of ways but the overall purpose is to ensure that each mentor:

- Has current knowledge of NMC-approved programmes.
- Is able to discuss the implications of changes to NMC requirements.
- Has the opportunity to discuss issues relating to mentoring, assessment of competence and fitness for safe and effective practice with others.

(NMC 2009:1)

How do I as a mentor provide evidence of updating?

You will need to demonstrate to your employer and also to NMC quality assurance agents (as appropriate) how you have maintained and developed your knowledge, skills and competence as a mentor. The employer as placement provider will review this evidence as part of an annual and/or triennial review which is explained in the following section.

For those mentors employed within the NHS in England, the NHS Knowledge and Skills Framework (NHS KSF) and development review process introduced by the Department of Health identifies that each employee must have an annual appraisal review and **personal development plan** agreed (DH 2004). Many Trusts have incorporated review of mentorship performance into this annual process. Where this has occurred, you will be enabled to develop and apply your knowledge and skills in meeting the demands of your role as mentor within your current post and to identify future learning and development needs.

Triennial review of mentors

Once mentors have been entered on the **local register** held by placement providers they must undergo a formal review at least every three years to remain 'live'. Placement providers can determine the nature of this review but whatever method is used, as already mentioned in Chapter 1, to be maintained on a local mentor register you must provide evidence of the following:

That you have:

- Mentored at least two students with due regard (extenuating circumstances permitting) within the three-year period.
- Participated in annual updating – this must include having met and explored assessment and supervision issues with other mentors/practice teachers.
- Explored as a group activity the validity and reliability of judgements made when assessing practice in challenging circumstances.
- Mapped ongoing development of your role against the current NMC mentor standards.
- Been deemed to have met all requirements needed to be maintained on the local register as a mentor or sign-off mentor.

(NMC 2008:12)

What is the practice placement responsibility in supporting mentors to update?

Continuing personal development (CPD) is a requirement for all mentors and the NMC standards (2008) reinforce the professional responsibilities of each practitioner to update within this role.

However, the employer also has an obligation to enable each practitioner to meet the requirements of his or her job role. Generally, at annual job evaluation/review meetings, a personal development plan (PDP) will be agreed, specifying the updating activities which will be supported by the employer.

If practitioners do not receive these opportunities and are, as a result, deemed not to have met the requirements to remain on the live mentor register they would have grounds to appeal through their employer's appeal process. The onus for CPD lies with each practitioner although any agreed and recorded development activities with a **reviewer** by means of the PDP (agreed at an annual job review meeting) should be honoured.

Government directives and UK health policy identified the importance of practice learning in *Making a Difference* (DH 1999) and directly influenced support for mentors in practice (Sharples *et al.* 2007). Mentors are tasked with the responsibility for all practice-based assessment decisions. The systems to support mentors in practice need to be robust, supportive and empowering for mentors. At the same time, the systems need to be able to ensure protection for patients by managing and where necessary 'failing' weak or poor performing students. As identified by Cassidy (2009: 39), mentors need to be 'conscious of providing safe, high quality patient care while supporting student participation and learning in complex care situations'. The appraisal/review process is an essential element in this process.

The appraisal/development review process

Performance appraisals are essential for the effective management and evaluation of staff performance. Organizational commitment to regular appraisal is built on the belief that:

- all members of staff have a right to a clear understanding of their manager's expectation of them;
- all members of staff have the right to an opportunity to discuss their contribution to the achievement of the ward/departmental goals; and
- appraisal offers the opportunity for staff to feel valued and to have their contribution acknowledged.

The appraisal process offers you as a mentor the opportunity to agree expectations and objectives, to review performance over a designated period and to identify and agree areas for future personal development by establishing individual training needs. For NMC mentors, who are required to demonstrate mentor competence on a three-yearly basis, part of their annual appraisal may involve a review of their performance as a mentor which is measured against some of the NMC mentor standards for the previous year, as agreed at a previous appraisal meeting. Thus, over a three-year period all of the NMC standards must be reviewed.

Appraisal review provides a formal, recorded review of an individual mentor's performance and a plan for future development. The appraisal review is a key process for identifying training and development needs of mentors and ensuring that they are met.

The appraisal review process aims to:

- ensure review of an individual's progress against agreed standards and objectives;

- identify an individual's strengths and development needs and facilitate discussions of personal aspirations (for example, a mentor may aspire to become a sign-off mentor);
- enhance the performance of the practice placement through assisting individual mentors to develop to their full potential.

The role of the reviewer in the appraisal/review process

It is the responsibility of all ward/department/service managers to ensure that all staff in their department or service are reviewed annually in line with their organization's appraisal policy. The appraiser and appraisee should agree a mutually convenient time to meet, so that both parties have sufficient time to prepare for the review meeting (see Chapter 5 for more detail on how a mentor could prepare for an appraisal). Specifically, time should be allocated and protected to ensure that the appraisal takes place and that neither the appraiser not the mentor being appraised is disturbed during the planned review process.

A mentor in clinical practice will be appraised by a named reviewer. This 'reviewer' may be their direct line manager or, alternatively, a named individual who has been delegated this responsibility by their direct line manager. The situation could arise that the appraiser is not a qualified mentor but he/she must clearly understand what is required before undertaking an appraisal or triennial review because the role of the reviewer is crucial in the process of making judgements about the competence of mentors. Appraisers will not normally review more than eight to ten individuals in any one year. Managers may therefore nominate alternative appraisers to perform the role of reviewer.

All appraisers/reviewers will normally have received appropriate training and preparation for the role.

This training will typically include:

- how to conduct a performance review;
- how to ensure that the process is robust;
- advice regarding the need to incorporate equality and diversity considerations during the review process. Appraisal/development reviews should not discriminate in any way on the grounds of gender, age, sexual orientation, race, religion or disability. The UK Employment Equality Regulations particularly stress that assessment cannot be based in any way on age-related factors (Employment Equality Regulations 2006).

Effective performance appraisal reviews

During the annual appraisal and/or triennial review, the reviewer will need to make judgements about whether you have demonstrated ongoing competence within your job role and also in your role as mentor/sign-off mentor. The NMC expect all mentors to map their ongoing development against the eight mentorship standards (NMC 2008). The judgements may be incorporated as part of a normal annual review meeting or may take place prior to the review itself, with confirmation of evidence being presented at review.

Preparing for the appraisal review

There are several things a line manager should do to prepare for an appraisal. These include:

- Prior to the review, the line manager should ensure that all reviewers have received appropriate training and are aware of the needs/standards required from a qualified mentor in practice; education providers and practice placement personnel may assist the line manager in this preparation.
- The reviewer should be familiar with the NMC standards to support learning and assessment in practice (2006, 2008) and all associated documentation which needs to be completed during the review.
- The reviewer should be aware of criteria on which to base his or her assessment. In particular, as with any performance appraisal process, care needs to be taken by the reviewer to consider the whole period under review, i.e. the past twelve months, and to base his or her assessment on the overall performance of the mentor during this period.
- The reviewer should aim to make the review a positive experience where he/she is seeking to help the mentor to develop fully as an individual. That is, not merely to identify relevant mentor knowledge and skills but, by supporting the development of the individual, to support positive attitudes and motivation so that the mentor can identify his or her potential to work more effectively.

To undertake a successful appraisal, the reviewer will need to consider the information listed above and also will need to prepare relevant material required to inform the discussion. This will usually include:

- a copy of the appraisee's job description which lists their responsibilities as a mentor;

- a copy of relevant NMC standards;
- individual records of previously agreed tasks or objectives;
- any additional information which pertains to the appraisee's performance or achievement over the assessment period;
- any records of incidents, awards or other relevant documentation.

The reviewer

At the annual review meeting, the reviewer will make judgements based on the evidence provided by the mentor, other reports or incidents which may have arisen during the annual period and discussions with the individual mentor.

Typically, the reviewer will review the activities, tasks, objectives and achievements one by one, keeping to distinct standards and criteria, concentrating on facts and solid evidence and avoiding anecdotal, non-specific conjecture or opinions. One of the most important criteria for a good reviewer is the need for objectivity. Reviewers must ensure that at all times they remain neutral and are not influenced by style, approach or image. Each standard should be considered by means of a measure of competence or achievement as relevant to the standard. Ideally, this should be identified by the organization as, for example, a scoring system built into the appraisal process. For example, performance can be scored against each objective (1 = unacceptable; 2 = satisfactory; 3 = good; 4 = excellent).

What happens at the appraisal?

At appraisal, you will produce evidence to support continuing professional development against two or three identified mentor standards for the previous 12 months. Alternatively, you may be required to produce evidence of annual updating and at triennial review to produce evidence to support continuing professional development against all eight domains of mentor competencies.

Whatever the local appraisal system agreed, the assessment of your ongoing competence as a mentor requires a judgement based on observation of a practitioner's performance against validated criteria of competence.

What criteria are used to judge whether a mentor has maintained ongoing competence?

These could include:

- evidence that they organize and co-ordinate student learning in practice;
- evidence of effective mentoring where the mentor encourages learners to manage their own learning;
- photocopies of documents showing that they have completed at least two student assessments during the period;
- examples of the way they challenge ideas and listen and communicate with others;
- relevant student evaluations;
- testimonials from peers or students;
- confirmation that the appraisee is listed on the local mentor register.

How would an appraiser rate mentorship performance?

In terms of making a judgement of the evidence produced, the appraiser may have agreed formal organizational **performance criteria**, or alternatively may need to develop their own set of criteria which they use consistently for all such assessments. The following table is an example of one such mentorship performance rating system.

Mentorship performance ratings

Excellent performance
This would be characterized by:
- exceeding the mentor objectives and standards set in terms of quantity and quality over a sustained period;
- fully meeting the mentor outline for the post and demonstrating some factors significantly above those required for the post;
- consistently role modelling organizational values and behaviours;
- consistently displaying, and empowering learners to adopt, the appropriate attitude in relation to service users, colleagues and other people they come in contact with in line with equality and diversity legislation.

Good performance
This would be characterized by:
- fully meeting the mentor objectives and standards set in terms of quantity and quality over a sustained period;
- fully meeting the mentor outline for the post and demonstrating some factors above those required for the post;

- consistently role modelling organizational values and behaviours and displaying, and empowering learners to adopt, the appropriate attitude in relation to service users, colleagues and other people they come in contact with in line with equality and diversity legislation.

Satisfactory performance
This would be characterized by:
- just meeting the mentor objectives and standards set in terms of quantity and quality;
- meeting the mentor outline for the post and demonstrating necessary progress towards fully meeting the post outline;
- displaying, and empowering learners to adopt, the appropriate attitude in relation to service users, colleagues and other people they come in contact with in line with equality and diversity legislation.

Unacceptable performance
This would be characterized by:
- failure to meet the objectives and standards set in terms of quantity and quality;
- not meeting the mentor outline for the post;
- displaying an inappropriate attitude in relation to service users, colleagues and other people they come in contact with in line with equality and diversity legislation;
- unacceptable professional practice.

What is being assessed at an appraisal?

As discussed in Chapter 2, pages 21–22, existing studies highlight the difficulties of ensuring validity and reliability of assessment tools which attempt to capture intangible aspects of nurses' competence such as attentiveness to patients and commitment (Norman *et al.* 2002; McMullan *et al.* 2003; Lofmark *et al.* 2006; Cassidy 2009). The situation is no different for reviewers when attempting to capture the performance of mentors themselves. Appraisal frameworks can assist reviewers in ensuring value-free assessment based on set performance criteria. This needs to be considered in the context of mentor behaviour and holistic assessment of competence.

The reviewer needs to take into account the following:

- the mentor's level of experience in the role;
- his or her level of confidence as an assessor.

The reviewer should also consider whether the support, training and development that has been provided by the mentor's manager, colleagues, practice development personnel and education providers has enabled the mentor to do his or her job effectively.

As part of the review process, the reviewer will discuss and agree with each mentor the skills, capabilities and experience required for competent performance in their current role. If appropriate, the reviewer will also explore the mentor's readiness to progress to the next role, for example progressing to the role of sign-off mentor. The reviewer will consider the connection between the mentor's personal talents, aspirations and work performance. Where additional opportunities or development opportunities are identified, the reviewer will seek to work with the mentor to identify relevant development opportunities and skills training to assist him or her to progress professionally and personally. This may include coaching, workshops, videos, reading, shadowing or distance learning.

During the review, the discussion between reviewer and mentor should also consider whether there have been any changes to the individual's job situation over the past year that have impacted on that person's ability to perform the role of mentor, such as changes to work patterns, staffing levels, or change of patient group. Any such issues should be documented.

Any valid assessment process must enable judgement to be made about the full range of required competencies in relation to the mandatory standards for mentorship. By adapting Wilcox and Brown's (2002) criteria that higher education institutions may use for assessing evidence presented in a portfolio, the following could be used during an appraisal interview:

- **Authenticity** – that the mentor really does what is claimed. What is the level of confidence that the mentor really does practise in the way that is evidenced in his or her portfolio? Is this backed up by direct observation, by feedback from colleagues and/or students?
- **Breadth** – that the learning/development was not isolated from wider dimensions e.g. service developments in place. The assessment of mentor competence requires a judgement based on a wider assessment of the mentor's ability to perform effectively in his or her professional role. Is there clear evidence that the overall performance of the mentor is adequate to make that person an acceptable role model in supervising and assessing more junior colleagues? Assessment based on real observation with/by other mentors, or by managers who have worked with the mentor over a continuous period has high face and content validity and is more robust in validating that competence is evidenced (McKinley *et al.* 2001).
- **Quality** – that the learning and development had reached an acceptable level congruent with the responsibilities of the job role. What is an 'acceptable quality level' will need to be determined locally and is beyond the remit of this book. However, consideration should be given to what activities the mentor has undertaken, what changes in performance have occurred as a result of this updating, and how this learning and development has been implemented in practice for the benefit of the individual, other learners, the placement area and the organization as a whole.
- **Currency** – that the mentor has kept up to date with recent developments. Evidence should be for the period being reviewed e.g. within the past 12 months for annual review and within the past three years for triennial review. Evidence provided which falls outside these parameters is normally not acceptable and not considered valid.

The reviewer will need to make an informed judgement based on the balance of written and verbal evidence provided by the mentor in the context of the opportunities available and support provided by the employer to demonstrate competence in the role, so it is essential that a mentor takes time to prepare and present this in a manner that clearly meets the requirements for maintaining his or her professional competence. If at the time of review this evidence has not been presented and the reviewer considers that this is insufficient reliable data on which to base a decision then the appraisal meeting should be rearranged and in exceptional circumstances deferred to a later date to allow the mentor time to produce the required evidence.

Chapter 5 provides further details on mapping learning to the NMC standards. It itemizes steps that can be undertaken following completion of **case study** which can be used by mentors to assist them in collating evidence of their learning for their professional portfolio and job appraisal.

At the formal review, the appraiser will confirm that after reviewing all evidence produced, he or she is assured that the practitioner has undertaken these activities and is competent/not competent to remain on the mentor register. If for any reason the appraiser records a decision of 'not competent' then reasons for this decision must be recorded on the appraisal/review documentation. An action plan will be agreed and all relevant parties notified of the decision. Both the mentor and appraiser will sign the completed form. One copy must remain with the mentor in his or her personal file, one copy will be retained by the appraiser and a copy will be forwarded to the relevant personnel to update the live mentor register.

Importantly, a system of recording can be undertaken to record the ongoing competence of mentors; examples of how this might be undertaken include:

- The live mentor register could be held by the human resource department or via an electronic system and accessed only by managers/appraisers.
- The system must be easily updatable, contain key information about mentors and their ongoing competence and be accessible to those who may need it e.g. managers, appraisers, educational providers (acknowledging data protection issues).
- The system must be able to record those who have successfully updated and maintained their ongoing competence, those who have not, those who are temporarily suspended and following an action plan and those who are sign-off mentors.
- The system must be sufficiently robust in linking to the appraisal system and any organizational appeal system if judgements about competence and fitness to fulfil a job role are reviewed.

Accountability obligations

Reviewers must have an in-depth understanding of their accountability to the NMC for the decisions that they make in regard to a mentor's ongoing competence. The difficulty of this has been previously discussed in Chapter 2, but the judgements in this instance should be made against locally agreed and national guidelines. A reviewer must be confident that the mentor demonstrates accountability by producing evidence that the requirements of the professional statutory regulatory body have been met. Further information on this may be obtained from an excellent article on accountability edited by Barnett (1997).

The role of the reviewer when mentors do not demonstrate ongoing competence in their role

Chapter 2 discussed the issue of 'competence' and identified the complexity involved with determining 'what level of performance indicates competence' and at what level an individual can be deemed 'incompetent'.

Situations may occur when a mentor does not demonstrate ongoing competence. This may include failure to provide sufficient, robust evidence on continuing development of skills, knowledge and competence against mentor standards at annual appraisal review. The following list provides examples of where this may occur:

- failure to maintain current registration status with the Nursing and Midwifery Council;
- failure to provide evidence against the agreed standards;
- failure to demonstrate how updating activities have been incorporated into their mentor role;
- failures to mentor at least two students with due regard (extenuating circumstances permitting) within the three-year period.

In these circumstances, the individual's appraiser/reviewer must inform the appropriate personnel depending on which roles exist within the organization. A learning and development plan will be agreed between the individual mentor and his or her manager, and a temporary suspension placed against the individual's name on the mentor register until competence has been satisfactorily demonstrated. If, following review, the individual mentor cannot demonstrate competence, and extenuating circumstances (such as long-term sick leave, career break) do not apply, consideration must be made by the appropriate personnel concerning permanent removal from the mentor register.

Summary

The aim of this chapter was to outline the organizational and reviewer requirements, from the practice placement provider perspective, in addressing the ongoing competence of mentors.

Key points

- Practice placement providers must maintain a live register of mentors and sign-off mentors.
- Practice placement providers are required to have relevant systems in place to monitor and update the live register, including adding or removing mentors' names.
- Performance appraisals are essential for the effective management and evaluation of staff performance.
- The appraisal process offers mentors the opportunity to agree expectations and objectives, to review performance over a designated period and to identify and agree areas for future personal development.
- The appraisal review is a key process for identifying training and development needs of mentors and ensuring that they are met.
- The assessment of mentor competence requires a judgement based on observation of a practitioner's performance against validated criteria of competence.
- Appraisal frameworks can assist reviewers in ensuring value-free assessment based on set performance criteria.
- As part of the review process, reviewers will discuss and agree with mentors the skills, capabilities and experience required for competent performance in their current role. If appropriate, they will also explore their readiness to progress to the next role, for example that of 'sign-off' mentor.
- Any valid assessment process must enable judgement to be made about the full range of required competencies. In relation to the mandatory standards for mentorship any such assessment should address 'authenticity', 'breadth', 'quality' and 'currency'.
- Reviewers must have an in-depth understanding of their accountability to the NMC for the decisions that they make in regard to a mentor's ongoing competence.

The next chapter will address each of the eight NMC standards. Through a case study approach, it will offer mentors the opportunity to explore each of the standards in detail and by working through a series of questions to develop and evidence their knowledge and skills as a mentor.

References

Barnett, D.E. (1997) *Sharing Information: Key Issues for the Nursing Professions*. The INFOrmed Touch Series, Volume 1. http://www.bcs.org/server.php?show=nav.10026 (Accessed 24 September 2009).

Cassidy, S. (2009) Interpretation of competence in student assessment, *Nursing Standard*, 23 (18): 39–46.

DBERR (Department for Business, Enterprise and Regulatory Reform) (2006) *Employment Equality (Age) Regulations*, SI 2006 No. 1031. London: DBERR.

DH (Department of Health) (1999) *Making a Difference: Strengthening the Nursing, Midwifery and Health Visiting Contribution to Health and Health Care*. London: Department of Health.

DH (2004) *The NHS Knowledge and Skills Framework (NHS KSF) and the Development Review Process*. London: Department of Health.

Lofmark, A., Smide, B. and Wilkblad, K. (2006) Competence of newly graduated nurses – a comparison of the preconceptions of qualified nurses and students, *Journal of Advanced Nursing*, 53 (6): 721–8.

McKinley, R.K., Fraser, R.C. and Baker, R. (2001) Model for directly assessing and improving clinical competence and performance in revalidation of clinicians, *British Medical Journal*, 322: 712–15 (24 March).

McMullan, M., Endacott, R., Gray, M., Jasper, K., Miller, C. and Webb, C. (2003) Portfolios and the assessment of competence: a review of the literature, *Journal of Advanced Nursing*, 41 (3): 283–94.

NMC (Nursing and Midwifery Council) (2006) *Standards to Support Learning and Assessment in Practice: NMC Standards for Mentors, Practice Teachers and Teachers*. London: NMC.

NMC (2007) *Applying Due Regard to Learning and Assessment in Practice*. http://www.nmc-uk.org/aDisplayDocument.aspx?documentID=3202 (Accessed 15 February 2010).

NMC (2008) *Standards to Support Learning and Assessment in Practice: NMC Standards for Mentors, Practice Teachers and Teachers*. London: NMC.

NMC (2009) *Additional Information to Support Implementation of NMC Standards to Support Learning and Assessment in Practice*. London: NMC.

Norman, I.J., Watson, R., Murrells, T., Calman, L. and Redfern, S. (2002) The validity and reliability of methods to assess the competence to practise of pre-registration nursing and midwifery students, *International Journal of Nursing Studies*, 39 (2): 133–45.

Sharples, K., Kelly, D. and Elcock, K. (2007) Supporting mentors in practice, *Nursing Standard*, 21(39): 44–7.

Wilcox, J. and Brown, R. (2002) *Accreditation of Prior and Experiential Learning – A Student Guide*. http://www.materials.ac.uk/resources/library/apelstudents.pdf (Accessed 22 December 2009).

Part 2

Mentorship Updating through Case Studies

4

Mentor Updating Using Case Studies

Lyn Rosen, Karen Staniland and Cyril Murray

Aim

The aim of this chapter is to enable you to develop and update your knowledge and skills as a mentor by working through case study materials, and to introduce the **case study section** of this book.

Learning outcomes

After reading this chapter you will be able to:

- recognize the link between the eight mandatory standards and the Knowledge and Skills Framework to promote and maintain your own ongoing competence;
- develop your knowledge and skills as a mentor using a range of case study materials;
- discuss with your peers a problem relating to the assessment of students to enhance the validity and reliability of judgments you will make as a mentor;
- identify the link between completing the case studies and assessment exercises as part of the appraisal process for maintaining your name on the live register of mentors.

Introduction

As a mentor there are many conflicting demands on your time which can affect your ability to support students (Wilkes 2006). However, the Nursing and Midwifery Council (NMC) clearly state in the *Standards to Support Learning and Assessment in Practice* (NMC 2008a) that all mentors are required to:

- participate in annual updating;
- map ongoing development against the eight mentorship standards.

As stated in Chapter 1, some mentors find it difficult to attend a traditional form of update, by presentation at a stipulated time, and would prefer some flexibility in how they update. The purpose of this chapter therefore is to offer you a new and exciting method of meeting the NMC requirements above, by using a **case study** approach.

The case studies featured in this book will enable you to explore in some detail each of the eight NMC standards. They require you to work through a series of questions relating to 'real' issues associated with mentoring. These derive from problem-based situations that have actually arisen in practice.

Completing the associated short exercises/activities will enable you to demonstrate how you are developing and maintaining your ongoing knowledge and competence, by recording your responses in your **professional development portfolio**.

You can also complement this activity in other ways which might include attendance at **workshops** held within your Trust/PCT or organized by the appropriate higher education institution.

The next sections explain the reasons why you should update and how to complete the update. You may also wish to refer to the NMC document *Standards to Support Learning and Assessment in Practice* (NMC 2008a).

Why do I need to update?

There are several reasons why both **mentors** and **registrants** should update on a regular basis and whilst we have covered this in other sections of this book, it is important to summarize the professional context in which the case studies sit. These include:

- The *Standards to Support Learning and Assessment in Practice* (NMC 2008a) and the subsequent document *Additional Information to Support Implementation of NMC Standards to Support Learning and Assessment in Practice* (NMC

2009) require mentors to maintain and develop their knowledge, skills and competence through annual updating.

- Under the Post-registration, Education and Practice (PREP) requirements (NMC 2008b) practitioners must maintain their ongoing competence within their professional role as a nurse, midwife and specialist community health practitioner. Evidence of continuing professional updating is a requirement when completing the renewal form for re-registering.

The NMC indicate that

Mentors and practice teachers must participate in **annual updating** – this is one of the requirements which they must meet in order to remain on the local register at triennial review. The annual updating process must include the opportunity to meet and explore assessment and supervision issues with other mentors/practice teachers (face-to-face) and explore as a group the **validity** and **reliability** of judgements made when assessing practice in challenging circumstances.

(NMC 2009: 3)

- Under the Code of Professional Conduct (NMC 2008c) it is a requirement of all practitioners to:

  ➢ keep their skills and knowledge up to date;
  ➢ facilitate students and others to develop their competence;
  ➢ deliver care based on the best available evidence or best practice.

- Under the *NHS Knowledge and Skills Framework* (KSF) (DH 2004) practitioners are required to have annual development reviews against their job outline. As part of this process personal development plans are agreed on how practitioners can work towards the role requirements of their job, which include being a mentor and/or associate mentor. The ultimate aim of the NHS KSF (DH 2004) is to provide safe, effective and quality healthcare.

The NMC state that to remain on the live register each individual practitioner must provide evidence of having:

- Mentored at least two students with due regard within the three-year period.
- Participated in annual updating – to include an opportunity to meet and explore assessment and supervision issues with other mentors/practice teachers.
- Explored as a group activity the validity and reliability of judgements made when assessing practice in challenging circumstances.
- Mapped ongoing development in their role against the current NMC mentor/practice teacher standards.

(NMC 2008a: 12)

What does the update consist of?

A case study has been developed for each of the eight mentorship standards and they are all included in this book.

Whilst you can update in several different ways to maintain your ongoing competence as a mentor, we are proposing that one way this can be achieved is through the completion of these case studies and a group assessment exercise each year.

By undertaking two/three case studies per year as part of annual updating you will have completed all eight standards after three years and be in a position to meet the requirements for your triennial review. This will contribute towards the maintenance of your place on the **live register** of mentors, in accordance with the Nursing and Midwifery Council (2008a) *Standards to Support Learning and Assessment in Practice*.

So, the completion of each case study will help you to:

- maintain your ongoing knowledge and skills to fulfil your role as a mentor;
- meet the requirements of your professional body;
- provide evidence as part of your personal development review with your employer;
- provide evidence of how you have maintained your ongoing competence in relation to your professional role. The standards could be agreed with your reviewer as part of an employer-led review under the NHS Knowledge and Skills Framework (DH 2004).

How will completing the case studies help me?

Each case study will help you to engage in problem solving, analysis, reflection and evaluation in order to develop your knowledge and future practice related to the associated standard. Evidence generated from the activities can be assembled in your professional development portfolio and can be used to demonstrate how you have maintained your ongoing knowledge and competence as a practising mentor in your practice area.

How do I complete the case studies?

- Review the NMC standards which you will find in the NMC *Standards to Support Learning and Assessment in Practice* (2008a).

- Identify the two/three standards you wish to focus on as part of your annual development, and choose the relevant case studies.
- Read the introduction to each case study. Read the case study and the relevant reading sources provided.
- Complete each question relating to each case study.
- Compare your responses with the suggestions provided in the Appendix (pages 115–140).
- If your responses are complete, move on to the next question.
- If your responses are incomplete, you are advised to revisit the recommended reading sources.
- Keep a copy of your work as a record of completion for your professional development portfolio.
- Map your learning from each case study to the specific standards.
- Identify appropriate evidence related to this activity to include in your professional development portfolio in preparation for your annual appraisal.

How do I complete the group assessment exercise?

- After you have completed the case studies, you are required to complete a group assessment exercise (NMC 2008a) – see case study nine. This is because the NMC (2008a) require you to engage in a group discussion with your peers on the validity and reliability of judgements concerned with assessment issues.
- After discussions with your peers, compare your responses with the suggested answers supplied.
- **We have included one example of an assessment exercise here but you will no doubt come across other real-time examples that you can discuss with your peers.**
- It will also be useful to provide information about the standards you have completed and the names of the practitioners who have engaged in the group discussion on the assessment exercise as a record for yourself and your workplace.

How do I map my learning to the NMC standards?

Complete the five steps below after you have completed each of the case studies. This will help you to collate evidence of your learning for your professional development portfolio or job appraisal. The steps involved require you to:

1 Identify the standards which are relevant to you e.g. NMC and the NHS KSF. The Health Professions Council (HPC) is not relevant here as the book is for nurse mentors.
2 Take each outcome or dimensional level within the standard and identify what resources you have used to address the standard arising from this case study.
3 Consider how this has been applied in your role as a mentor.
4 Reflect upon what you have learnt from these experiences.
5 Identify what evidence you can provide to demonstrate your learning and development as a mentor from the above steps.

How do I update my name on the live register?

By completing two/three case studies within one year and providing evidence to your appraiser you will now be in a position to complete the annual update form (or its equivalent). This information will then need to be forwarded to the person within your Trust/PCT who maintains the live register of mentors.

References

DH (Department of Health) (2004) *The NHS Knowledge and Skills Framework and Development Review Process*. http://www.dh.gov.uk/en/Publicationsandstatistics/Publications/PublicationsPolicyAndGuidance/DH_4090843 (Accessed 14 September 2009).

NMC (Nursing and Midwifery Council) (2008a) *Standards to Support Learning and Assessment in Practice: NMC Standards for Mentors, Practice Teachers and Teachers*. http://www.nmc-uk.org/aDisplayDocument.aspx?documentID=4368 (Accessed 10 July 2009).

NMC (2008b) *The Prep Handbook*. http://www.nmc-uk.org/aDisplayDocument. aspx?documentID=4340 (Accessed 14 September 2009).

NMC (2008c) *The Code: Standards of Conduct, Performance and Ethics for Nurses and Midwives*. http://www.nmc-uk.org/aArticle.aspx?ArticleID=3056 (Accessed 14 September 2009).

NMC (2009) *Additional Information to Support Implementation of NMC Standards to Support Learning and Assessment in Practice*. http://www.nmc-uk.org/aDisplayDocument. aspx?documentID=5653 (Accessed 14 September 2009).

Wilkes, Z. (2006) The student–mentor relationship: a review of the literature, *Nursing Standard*, 20(37): 42–7.

Case Studies

The following section of this chapter will take you through the eight manda-tory standards. Follow the instructions outlined on the previous pages to help you complete them. In summary:

- Review the relevant NMC standard.
- Read the introduction to the case study.
- Read the case study carefully and then, taking each question in turn, record your answers in your professional development portfolio.
- Go to the relevant page in the Appendix to compare your responses to those suggested.
- Consider expanding your responses after reading these.

You will notice that we have not given an estimated time for completion of the questions. This is because we recognize that mentors are individuals and, depending on their experience and required reading, some may need further periods of reflection than others in order to complete these. We would recommend, if you do think that you are taking more time than you feel is justifiable, that you consult your colleagues or turn the question into a group exercise. Alternatively you could contact your higher education establishment for advice.

Case Study 1

Establishing Effective Working Relationships

Before commencing on this case study it is important for you to have reviewed the Nursing and Midwifery Standard for Establishing Effective Working Relationships in Practice.

This case study offers you the opportunity to explore how establishing effective working relationships can influence practice. It can be analysed and reflected upon individually or discussed with peers in a group situation. It specifically relates to the NMC Standard: Establishing Effective Working Relationships.

The outcomes for this standard are:

- Demonstrate an understanding of factors that influence how students integrate into practice settings.
- Provide ongoing and constructive support to facilitate transition from one learning environment to another.
- Have effective professional and inter-professional working relationships to support learning for entry to the register.

(NMC 2008: 20)

This case study has also been mapped to the NHS KSF (DH 2004), which consists of a range of **core** and specific **dimensions** that describe the knowledge and skills that mentors will need to apply in their job role. It relates specifically to the following:

Core dimensions 1 to 6

Specific dimensions

- IK1 – Information Processing
- IK2 – Information Collection and Analysis

- IK3 – Knowledge and Information Resources
- G1 – Learning and Development
- G6 – People Management

Case study

You are mentoring Dawn, a third-year student nurse who is completing her final placement prior to qualification. She is in Week 4 of her placement. Dawn is concerned that, apart from her community placement in the second year where she was attached to a district nurse who ran a leg ulcer clinic, she has had very little experience of dealing with the multi-professional team and outside agencies.

You are anxious that Dawn should have a good understanding of the importance of developing relationships with other departments both within and outside the hospital, and have therefore suggested that she helps with the organization of a multi-professional team meeting for a patient who has complex needs. This patient has a number of internal and external agencies already involved in the care plan. The student has asked for your opinion on how best to contact and establish a relationship with those who have been invited to the meeting.

Key questions

Below are a series of questions related to the case study. Read the questions carefully and then write your responses in your professional development portfolio. After this, compare your answers with the suggestions on pages 115–118.

1 What are the main issues arising from this case study?
2 How are effective working relationships maintained?
3 What do you have to do to facilitate Dawn's learning in relation to establishing working relationships?
4 What would Dawn's involvement entail?
5 What boundaries, if any, need to be in place?
6 What might be the barriers to effective inter-professional working?
7 What strategies could Dawn utilize to overcome these barriers?
8 What is her professional responsibility?
9 What competencies/skills are **transferable** from this case study?

Possible sources of materials to inform your knowledge and practice

DH (Department of Health) (1994) *Working in Partnership: A Collaborative Approach to Care* (Report of Mental Health Nursing Review Team). London: Department of Health.

DH (1996) *Building Collaborative Links: Partnerships in Care*. London: Department of Health.

DH (1998) *Working Together: Securing a Quality Workforce for the NHS*. London: Department of Health.

DH (1999) *Health Act Partnership Arrangements*. London: Department of Health.

DH (2004) *The NHS Knowledge and Skills Framework (NHS KSF) and the Development Review Process*. London: Department of Health.

Fakhoury, W.K.H. and Wright, D. (2000) Communication and information needs of a random sample of community psychiatric nurses in the United Kingdom, *Journal of Advanced Nursing*, 32 (4): 871–80.

Farrell, M.P., Schmitt, M.H. and Heinemann, G.D. (2001) Informal roles and the stages of interdisciplinary team development, *Journal of Interprofessional Care*, 15 (3): 281–95.

Freeman, M., Miller, C. and Ross, N. (2000) The impact of individual philosophies of teamwork on multi-professional practice and the implications for education, *Journal of Interprofessional Care*, 14 (3): 237–47.

Glendinning, C. (2002) Breaking down barriers: integrating health and care services for older people in England, *Health Policy*, 65: 139–51.

Gribben, B. and Cochrane, C. (2006) Critical companionship: our learning journey, *Practice Developments in Health Care*, 5(1): 14–19.

Henwood, M. and Hudson, B. (2000) *Partnership and the NHS Plan: Cooperation or Coercion? The Implications for Social Care*. Leeds: Nuffield Institute for Health.

Hudson, B. (2002) Interprofessionality in health and social care: the Achilles' heel of partnership?, *Journal of Interprofessional Care*, 16 (1): 7–17.

Leathard, A. (ed.) (2003) *Interprofessional Collaboration: From Policy to Practice in Health and Social Care*. London: Brunner Routledge.

McNeal, M., Oster, R. and Alema-Mensah, E. (1999) Health professions students' opinions of interdisciplinary health care teams, *National Academies of Practice Forum*, 1 (1): 17–23.

Nursing and Midwifery Council (2008) *Standards to Support Learning and Assessment in Practice: NMC Standards for Mentors, Practice Teachers and Teachers*. London: NMC.

Ovretveit, J., Mathias, P. and Thompson, T. (eds) (1997) *Interprofessional Working for Health and Social Care*. Basingstoke: Macmillan.

Phelan, A.M., Barlow, C.A. and Iversen, S. (2006) Occasioning learning in the workplace: the case of interprofessional peer collaboration, *Journal of Interprofessional Care*, 20(4): 415–24.

Salmon, D. and Jones, M. (2001) Shaping the interprofessional agenda: a study examining qualified nurses' perceptions of learning with others, *Nurse Education Today*, 21: 18–25.

Tracey, C. and Nicholl, H. (2006) Mentoring and networking, *Nursing Management UK*, 12(10): 28–32.

Journals

Journal of Interprofessional Care
Journal of Advanced Nursing

Organizations

CAIPE http://www.caipe.org.uk (Accessed 17 September 2009).
Dedicated to the promotion and development of inter-professional education (IPE) with and through its individual and corporate members, in collaboration with like-minded organizations in the UK and overseas. It provides information and advice through its website, bulletins, papers and outlets provided by others, and has a close association with the *Journal of Interprofessional Care.*

Department of Health http://www.dh.gov.uk (Accessed 17 September 2009).
Providing health and social care policy, guidance and publications for NHS and social care professionals.

King's Fund http://www.kingsfund.org.uk/ (Accessed 17 September 2009).
A charitable foundation in England. It seeks to understand how the health system in England can be improved. Using that insight, it helps to shape policy, transform services and bring about behaviour change. Its work includes research, analysis, leadership development and service improvement. It also offers a wide range of resources to help everyone working in health to share knowledge, learning and ideas.

Nursing and Midwifery Council http://www.nmc-uk.org (Accessed 17 September 2009).
Exists to safeguard the health and well-being of the public.

Procare http://www.euro.centre.org/procare/ (Accessed 17 September 2009).
An organization which is helping to define the new concept of integrated health and social care for the needs of older people. It compares and evaluates different models. Some reports are available online or by emailing the project leads.

Case Study 2

Facilitation of Learning

Before commencing on this case study it is important for you to have reviewed the NMC Standard for Facilitation of Learning.

This case study offers you the opportunity to explore how you as a mentor can facilitate student learning. It can be analysed and reflected upon individually or discussed with peers in a group situation. It specifically relates to the NMC Standard: Facilitation of Learning.

The outcomes for this standard are:

- Use knowledge of the student's stage of learning to select appropriate learning opportunities to meet individual needs.
- Facilitate the selection of appropriate learning strategies to integrate learning from practice and academic experiences.
- Support students in critically reflecting upon their learning experiences in order to enhance future learning.

(NMC 2008: 20)

This case study has also been mapped to the NHS KSF (DH 2004), which consists of a range of core and specific dimensions that describe the knowledge and skills that mentors will need to apply in their job role. It relates specifically to the following:

Core dimensions

- Core Dimension 4 – Service Improvement
- Core Dimension 5 – Quality

Specific dimensions

- HWB5 – Provision of Care to Meet Health and Well Being Needs
- HWB7 – Plan, Deliver and Evaluate Interventions and/or Treatment
- G1 – Learning and Development

Case study

Student nurse Joanne Forester is allocated to your clinical area for semester 1 of year 3 on her pre-registration programme. Joanne has been involved with other members of the health care team in heated verbal interactions over miscommunication about patients' dietary needs and incorrect moving and handling of a patient.

Joanne, who is not averse to expressing her personal views, has commented to other staff that she has no time for other healthcare professionals whom she perceives are 'visitors' to the ward.

As her mentor you are about to do her intermediate interview. As part of her practice assessment she is required to develop effective inter-professional working practices that respect and utilize the contributions of members of the health and social care team.

Key questions

Below are a series of questions related to the case study. Read the questions carefully and then write your responses in your professional development portfolio. After this compare your answers with the suggestions on pages 119–120.

1 What are the key issues arising from this case study?
2 How could you as a mentor facilitate Joanne's learning needs during her placement?
3 What steps can you take as a mentor to ensure that your knowledge and practice on the facilitation of learning is current?
4 What steps can you take to ensure that Joanne's learning needs are facilitated in your absence?

Possible sources of materials to inform your knowledge and practice

Barr, H. (2002) *Interprofessional Education Today, Yesterday and Tomorrow: A Review*. Learning and Teaching Support Network for Health Sciences and Practice. London: CAIPE.

Dickinson, E. and Deighan, M. (1999) Editorial collaboration and communication – the millennium agenda for clinical improvement?, *International Journal for Quality in Health Care*, 11: 279–81.

Dickinson, C., Walker, J. and Bourgeois, S. (2006) Facilitating undergraduate nurses' clinical practicum. The lived experience of clinical facilitators, *Nurse Education Today*, 26(5): 416–22.

DH (Department of Health) (1996) *In the Patient's Interest: Multi-professional Working Across Organisational Boundaries*. London: DH.

DH (1998) *New Opportunities for Joint Working Between Health and Social Services: Strategic Planning, Service Commissioning and Service Provision*. London: DH.

DH (2001) *Making the Change: A Strategy for Professions in Healthcare Science*. London: DH.

DH (2002) *Learning Disabilities: Good Practice Guidance on Partnership Working*. London: DH

DH (2003) *Learning for Collaborative Practice with Other Professions and Agencies: A Study to Inform Development of the Degree in Social Work*. London: DH.

DH (2004a) *Making it Happen. Chapter 6 in NHS Improvement Plan: Putting People at the Heart of Public Services*. London: DH.

DH (2004b) *Making Partnership Work for Patients, Carers and Service Users: A Strategic Agreement Between the Department of Health, the NHS and the Voluntary and Community Sector*. London: DH.

DH (2004c) *The NHS Knowledge and Skills Framework (NHS KSF) and the Development Review Process*. London: DH.

HPC (Health Professions Council) (2003) *Standards of Conduct, Performance and Ethics*. London: HCP.

HPC (2005) *Standards of Education and Training*. London: HCP.

Krogstad, U., Hofoss, D. and Hjortdahl, P. (2004) Doctor and nurse perception of inter-professional co-operation in hospitals, *International Journal for Quality in Health Care*, 16(6): 491–7.

NMC (Nursing and Midwifery Council) (2004a) *Standards of Proficiency for Pre-registration Nursing Education*. http://www.nmc-uk.org/aFrameDisplay.aspx?DocumentID=328 (Accessed 23 September 2009).

NMC (2004b) *Standards of Proficiency for Pre-registration Midwifery Education*. http://www.nmc-uk.org/aFrameDisplay.aspx?DocumentID=171 (Accessed 15 September 2009).

NMC (2008) *Code of Professional Conduct, Standards for Conduct, Performance and Ethics*. London: NMC.

Nursing and Midwifery Council (2008) *Standards to Support Learning and Assessment in Practice: NMC Standards for Mentors, Practice Teachers and Teachers*. London: NMC.

Saarikoski, M., Warne, T. and Leino-Kilpi, H. (2006) Group supervision in facilitating learning in mental health clinical placement. A case example of one student group, *Issues in Mental Health Nursing*, 27(3): 273–85.

United Kingdom Central Council (1999) *Fitness for Practice*. Report by UKCC Commission for Nursing and Midwifery Education, Chaired by Sir Leonard Peach. http://www.nmc-uk.org/aFrameDisplay.aspx?DocumentID=627 (Accessed 15 September 2009).

Case Study 3

Assessment and Accountability

Before commencing this case study it is important for you to have reviewed the Nursing and Midwifery Standard for Assessment and Accountability.

This case study offers you the opportunity to explore how you as a mentor are accountable for the assessment of student learning. It examines the issues surrounding a failing student and can be analysed and reflected upon individually or discussed with peers in a group situation. It specifically relates to the NMC Standard: Assessment and Accountability.

The outcomes for this standard are:

- Foster professional growth, personal development and accountability through support of students in practice.
- Demonstrate a breadth of understanding of assessment strategies and the ability to contribute to the total assessment process as part of the teaching team.
- Provide constructive feedback to students and assist them in identifying future learning needs and actions. Manage failing students so that they may either enhance their performance and capabilities for safe and effective practice or be able to understand their failure and the implications of this for their future.
- Be accountable for confirming that students have met, or not met, the NMC competencies in practice. As a sign-off mentor confirm that students have met, or not met the NMC standards of proficiency in practice and are capable of safe and effective practice.

(NMC 2008a: 20)

This case study has also been mapped to the NHS KSF (DH 2004), which consists of a range of core and specific dimensions that describe the knowledge and skills that mentors will need to apply in their job role. It relates specifically to the following:

Core dimensions 1 to 6

Specific dimensions

- IK1 – Information Processing
- IK2 – Information Collection and Analysis
- IK3 – Knowledge and Information Resources
- G1 – Learning and Development
- G6 – People Management

Case study

James is a first-year student who is coming to the end of his first placement experience. He previously had been a healthcare assistant for three years before deciding to embark upon nursing as a career. He has a reputation of being a cocky but confident individual who enjoys showing others what he can do.

James is undertaking an eight-week experience on a medical placement on a different ward on which he had previously worked within the Trust as a healthcare assistant. The practice assessment is summative in nature and Susan, his nominated mentor, went off on long-term sick after he had been on the ward three weeks. Some of the clinical staff have been concerned about James's behaviour to them and to the patients. He is reported to have answered senior clinical members back, observed to have shouted at a patient who would not get out of bed and undertaken clinical activities such as changing an intravenous infusion bag without permission or supervision by a qualified staff member. He had been allowed to change infusion bags previously as a healthcare assistant.

These individual incidents were not addressed at the time at which they occurred but were reported to his mentor (Susan) who had intended to raise them at his midpoint interview but went off sick before this could occur. A new mentor called Joanna was appointed on Week 5 but due to excessive workload pressures on the ward a midpoint interview was not carried out. James's behaviour continued as before.

On Week 8 Joanna met with James for his final interview. He believed the placement had gone well and that he had achieved his outcomes of learning as required on the practice assessment document. Joanna felt otherwise and informed James that he had failed his placement assessment on two areas:

- his professional behaviour was poor;
- he undertook care management/delivery activities without permission.

However, no evidence was produced at the final interview and the documentation only made reference to his attitude being inappropriate for a nurse.

Key questions

Below are a series of questions related to the case study. Read the questions carefully and then write your responses in your professional development portfolio. After this compare your answers with the suggestions on pages 120–123.

1 What are the key issues arising from this case study?
2 Has James received a fair assessment?
3 What are the requirements for a fair assessment?
4 What evidence should have been collected from this case study?
5 How could James's assessment have been formally documented?
6 What rights has James in relation to this assessment?
7 What are the legal and ethical implications for the mentor in relation to this case study?
8 What should have been undertaken differently by the mentor and the ward team in relation to supporting and assessing James?
9 What quality assurance implications arise from this case study?

Possible sources of materials to inform your knowledge and practice

Burgess, R., Phillips, R. and Skinner, K. (1998) Practice placements that go wrong, *Journal of Practice Teaching*, 1(2): 48–64.

DH (Department of Health) (2004) *The NHS Knowledge and Skills Framework (NHS KSF) and Development Review Process*. London: Department of Health.

Dimond, B. (2002) Getting it right: the legal and professional aspects of assessment, in I. Welsh and C. Swann, *Partners In Learning: A Guide to Support and Assessment in Nurse Education*. Oxford: Radcliffe Medical Press.

Dolan, G. (2003) Assessing student nurse clinical competency. Will we ever get it right?, *Journal of Clinical Nursing*, 12: 132–41.

Duffy, K. (2003) *Failing Students: A Qualitative Study of Factors that Influence the Decisions Regarding Assessment of Students' Competence in Practice*. http://www.york.ac.uk/healthsciences/mentors/failingstudents.pdf (Accessed 15 September 2009).

NMC (Nursing and Midwifery Council) (2008a) *Standards of Conduct, Performance and Ethics for Nurses and Midwives*. London: NMC.

Nursing and Midwifery Council (2008b) Standards to Support Learning and Assessment in Practice: NMC Standards for Mentors, Practice Teachers and Teachers. London: NMC.

Scanlon, J., Care, W. and Gessler, S. (2001) Dealing with the unsafe student in clinical practice, *Nurse Educator*, 26(1): 23–7.

Sharp, M. (2000) The assessment of incompetence: practice teachers' support needs when working with failing DipSW students, *Journal of Practice Teaching*, 2(3): 5–18.

Stuart, C. (2003) *Assessment, Supervision and Support in Clinical Practice*. Edinburgh: Churchill Livingstone.

Case Study 4

Evaluation of Learning

Before commencing on this case study it is important for you to have reviewed the Nursing and Midwifery Standard for Evaluation of Learning.

This case study offers you the opportunity to explore how the mentor can contribute to the evaluation of student learning. It can be analysed and reflected upon individually or discussed with peers in a group situation. It specifically relates to the NMC Standard: Evaluation of Learning.

The outcomes for this standard are:

- Contribute to evaluation of student learning and assessment experiences – proposing aspects for change resulting from such evaluation.
- Participate in self and peer evaluation to facilitate personal development, and contribute to the development of others.

(NMC 2008: 20)

This case study has also been mapped to the NHS KSF (DH 2004), which consists of a range of core and specific dimensions that describe the knowledge and skills that mentors will need to apply in their job role. It relates specifically to the following:

Core dimensions 1 to 6

Specific dimensions

- IK1 – Information Processing
- IK2 – Information Collection and Analysis
- IK3 – Knowledge and Information Resources
- G1 – Learning and Development
- G6 – People Management

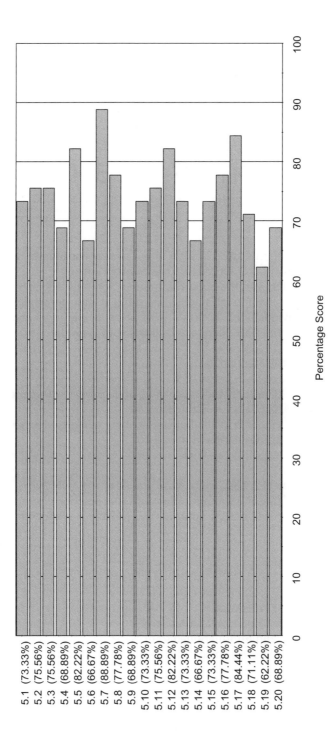

Percentage Score

Figure 4.1 Nine student responses of evaluation of practice

5.1 Teaching and learning are seen as important.
5.2 Staff are willing to teach.
5.3 Students are encouraged to ask questions.
5.4 Learning needs are recognized and help is given with the learning outcomes/action plans.
5.5 Helpful orientation is provided for the students at the start of the placement/within the first 24 hours.
5.6 Students are introduced to their mentor/associate mentor within the first 24 hours of being on the placement.
5.7 Students work with their mentor/associate mentors at least two shifts per week.
5.8 Assessment interviews are conducted at the appropriate times i.e. initial, intermediate and final.
5.9 Students remain supernumerary.
5.10 Students are given regular feedback on progress.
5.11 All qualified staff are engaged in care delivery/service.
5.12 Students are actively encouraged to observe/undertake new activities commensurate with their stage in training.
5.13 Students are encouraged (under supervision) to contribute to individual care plans.
5.14 There are up-to-date learning resources (books, journals, articles, IT) available for student use.
5.15 Students have opportunities to work with members of the multidisciplinary team.
5.16 Students are given the opportunity to follow care via a variety of pathways.
5.17 Evidence-based care is practised.
5.18 All students' learning experiences with other members of the placement team are guided by their mentor.
5.19 Students are made to feel welcome and part of the team.
5.20 Good communications exist to facilitate the delivery of care.

Case study

The evaluation form (see pages 68–69) has been forwarded to the placement. The percentage score is the level of student satisfaction with the said statement. The graph represents a cumulative score for each of the statements on the attached evaluation form (based on the number of students who have completed a placement allocation). The maximum achievable for a said statement is 100 per cent. If the graph line extends beyond half way (50 per cent) on the axis, then the placement is acceptable in terms of that statement, but further developmental work may be required and an action plan must be completed. You have been shown this form by the **Placement Educational Lead** (PEL) who is seeking your views on how to address the low scores and improve the overall placement experience for the students.

Key questions

Below are a series of questions related to the case study. Read the questions carefully and then write your responses in your professional development portfolio. After this compare your answers with the suggestions on pages 124–126.

1 What are the main issues arising from this case study?
2 Whose responsibility is it to resolve the issues arising from this evaluation?
3 What needs to be undertaken as a result of this evaluation?
4 What additional resources can you draw upon to support the changes you are suggesting/making in order to convince your peers?
5 The student evaluation identified that some current practices need to change. What change management approach/theoretical model could you propose to the PEL which might assist this process?
6 A culture needs to be created within the clinical area that embeds a commitment by all practitioners towards self and peer evaluation processes. What steps could be taken to achieve this?

Possible sources of materials to inform your knowledge and practice

Beitler, M. (2006) *Strategic Organizational Change*, 2nd edn. Greensboro, NC: Practitioner Press International.

Bennet, C. and Ferlie, E. (1994) *Managing Crisis and Change in Healthcare*. Milton Keynes: Open University Press.

DH (Department of Health) (2004) *The NHS Knowledge and Skills Framework (NHS KSF) and the Development Review Process*. London: DH.

Drennan, J. (2002) An evaluation of the role of the clinical placement coordinator in student nurse support in the clinical area, *Journal of Advanced Nursing*, 40 (4): 475–83.

Drucker, P. (1981) *Management in Turbulent Times*. London: Pan.

Fakhoury, W.K.H. and Wright, D. (2000) Communication and information needs of a random sample of community psychiatric nurses in the United Kingdom, *Journal of Advanced Nursing*, 32 (4): 871–80.

Gilmour, J.A. (2007) Student nurses as peer-mentors: collegiality in practice, *Nurse Education in Practice*, 71: 36–43.

Guba, E. and Lincoln, E.S. (1981) *Effective Evaluation*. San Francisco, CA: Jossey Bass.

Handy, C. (1990) *Inside Organisations*. London: BBC Books.

Harward, L.M. (2000) Becoming a self-reflective teacher: a meaningful research process, *Journal of Physical Therapy Education*, 14 (1): 21–30.

Hixenbaugh, P., Dewart, H., Drees, D. and Williams, D. (2005) Peer e-mentoring: enhancement of the first year experience, *Psychology Learning and Teaching*, 5 (1): 8–14.

Lewin, K. (1951) *Field Theory in Social Science*. New York: Harper and Row.

NMC (Nursing and Midwifery Council) (2008) *Standards to Support Learning and Assessment in Practice: NMC Standards for Mentors, Practice Teachers and Teachers*. London: NMC.

Plant, R. (1987) *Managing Change and Sticking To It*. London: Fontana.

Rogers, A. (2000) How can we tell . . ., in C.M. Downie and P. Basford (eds), *Teaching and Assessing in Clinical Practice: A Reader*. London: University of Greenwich.

Rogers, E.M. (2003) *Diffusion of Innovation*. New York: Free Press.

Ronsten, B. (2005) Confirming mentorship, *Journal of Nursing Management*, 13 (4): 312–21.

Rosser, M. (2004) Evaluation of a mentorship programme for specialist practitioners, *Nurse Education Today*, 24 (8): 596–604.

Spurgeon, P. and Barwell, F. (1991) *Implementing Change in the NHS*. London: Chapman and Hall.

Tracey, C. and Nicholl, H. (2006) Mentoring and networking, *Nursing Management UK*, 12: 1028–32.

Wilson, D.C. and Rosenfeld, R.H. (1990) *Managing Organisations*. London: McGraw-Hill.

Worren, N.A.M., Ruddle, K. and Moore, K. (1999) From organizational development to change management: the emergence of a new profession, *Journal of Applied Behavioural Science*, 35 (3): 273–86.

Case Study 5

Creating an Environment for Learning

Before commencing on this case study it is important for you to have reviewed the Nursing and Midwifery Standard for Creating an Environment for Learning.

This case study offers you the opportunity to explore how creating an environment for learning can influence student learning. It can be analysed and reflected upon individually or discussed with peers in a group situation. It specifically relates to the following NMC Standard: Creating an Environment for Learning.

The outcomes for this standard are:

- Support students to identify both learning needs and experiences appropriate to their level of learning.
- Use a range of learning experiences, involving patients, clients, carers and the professional team, to meet defined learning needs.
- Identify aspects of the learning environment which could be enhanced – negotiating with others to make appropriate changes.
- Act as a resource to facilitate personal and professional development of others.

(NMC 2008: 20)

This case study has also been mapped to the NHS KSF (DH 2004), which consists of a range of core and specific dimensions that describe the knowledge and skills that mentors will need to apply in their job role. It relates specifically to the following:

Core dimensions 1 to 6

Specific dimensions

- IK1 – Information Processing
- IK2 – Information Collection and Analysis
- IK3 – Knowledge and Information Resources
- G1 – Learning and Development
- G6 – People Management

Case study

Amy Jones is a Staff Nurse who works on a 32-bedded general medical ward in a large inner city hospital. She has been an **associate mentor** for six years and is currently studying for the mentorship qualification. The ward regularly has nursing students placed there and has a capacity for three students to be on placement at a time. The ward usually operates at its capacity for students, who range from first to third years. There are two other mentors working on the ward and one other associate mentor.

The previous two student evaluations have indicated that some improvements could be made with regards to the learning environment of the ward. Specifically, reference was made to the lack of learning resources available to students and the limited opportunities students have to work with other members of the multi-disciplinary team. A deficit was also highlighted in the opportunities provided for students to identify their own individual learning needs and in the support provided in accessing learning experiences to meet those needs.

The ward manager has asked Staff Nurse Jones to examine strategies for improving the learning environment and produce a series of recommendations. These recommendations will be reviewed in partnership by the staff and management on the ward and university representatives.

Key questions

Below are a series of questions related to the case study. Read the questions carefully and then write your responses in your professional development portfolio. After this compare your answers with the suggestions on pages 126–129.

1 What are the key issues arising from this case study?
2 What support and resources should Amy access to help her with this task?

3 Why is it important that students are able to identify their own learning needs?
4 What processes exist to help students identify their learning needs and what is the mentor's role in relation to this?
5 Give four examples of learning resources that could be provided to support students and staff development in this clinical area?
6 How can Amy support the other staff on the ward to ensure that students' learning needs are effectively met in a safe environment?
7 Why is it important for students to experience working with members of the multi-professional team?
8 How can Amy provide opportunities for **inter-professional learning**?
9 What strategies could Amy develop to continuously monitor the quality of the learning environment?

Possible sources of materials to inform your knowledge and practice

DH (Department of Health) (2004) *The NHS Knowledge and Skills Framework (NHS KSF) and the Development Review Process*. London: DH.

ENB (English National Board) and DH (Department of Health) (2001) *Placements in Focus: Guidance for Education in Practice for Health Care Professions*. London: ENB DH.

Hand, H. (2006) Promoting effective teaching and learning in the clinical setting, *Nursing Standard*, 20 (39): 55–63.

Hart, G. and Rotem, A. (1995) The clinical learning environment: nurses' perceptions of professional development in clinical settings, *Nurse Education Today*, 15(1): 3–10.

Nicklin, P. (2000) The learning environment, in P. Nicklin and N. Kenworthy (eds) *Teaching and Assessing in Nursing Practice*, 3rd edn. London: Balliere Tindall.

NMC (Nursing and Midwifery Council) (2008) *Standards to Support Learning and Assessment in Practice: NMC Standards for Mentors, Practice Teachers and Teachers*. London: NMC.

Price, B. (2004a) Building your learning environment, *Nursing Standard*, 19(9).

Price, B. (2004b) Evaluating your learning environment, *Nursing Standard*, 19(5).

Price, B. (2005) Liaising with the university, *Nursing Standard*, 20(9).

QAA (Quality Assurance Agency for Higher Education) (2001) *Code of Practice for Placement Learning*. London: QAA.

Royal College of Nurses (RCN) (2007) *Guidance for Mentors of Student Nurses and Midwives: An RCN Toolkit*. London: RCN.

Stuart, C. (2003) *Assessment, Supervision and Support in Clinical Practice: A Guide for Nurses, Midwives and Other Health Professionals*. London: Churchill Livingstone.

Thompson, S. (2003) Creating a learning environment, in S. Hinchliff (ed.) *The Practitioner as a Teacher*, 3rd edn. London: Churchill Livingstone.

Case Study 6

Context of Practice

Before commencing on this case study it is important for you to have reviewed the Nursing and Midwifery Standard for the Context of Practice.

This case study offers you the opportunity to explore how the context of professional practice can influence student learning. It can be analysed and reflected upon individually or discussed with peers in a group situation. It specifically relates to the NMC Standard: Context of Practice.

The outcomes for this standard are:

- Contribute to the development of an environment in which effective practice is fostered, implemented, evaluated and disseminated.
- Set and maintain professional boundaries that are sufficiently flexible for providing inter-professional care.
- Initiate and respond to practice developments to ensure safe and effective care is achieved and an effective learning environment is maintained.

(NMC 2008: 20/21)

This case study has also been mapped to the NHS KSF (DH 2004), which consists of a range of core and specific dimensions that describe the knowledge and skills that mentors will need to apply in their job role. It relates specifically to the following:

Core dimensions 1 to 6

Specific dimensions

- IK1 – Information Processing
- IK2 – Information Collection and Analysis
- IK3 – Knowledge and Information Resources
- G1 – Learning and Development
- G6 – People Management.

Case study

This case study, although specifically referring to a child branch student, can be applied to any pre-registration student.

Kelsey is a child branch student who is half way through her first nine-week placement in her third year. She has progressed steadily through the programme, achieving pass grades in the low forties, and has successfully completed all practice assessments. Her previous practice mentor noted that Kelsey has a quiet disposition. She works hard on the ward but rarely asks questions.

Kelsey is now working on a busy children's surgical ward. On this particular day she had been allocated the care of three children by her mentor. Her mentor is in charge of the ward. Two were recovering from minor surgery and were due to be discharged that day. The third child, a 5-year-old girl, Shona, was scheduled for theatre later that morning. Shona had been receiving intravenous fluids but this had been stopped because the cannula had ceased to function properly.

Soon after the shift began a doctor approached Kelsey and told her that he needed to site an intravenous cannula in Shona so she could receive intravenous fluids before going to theatre.

Kelsey prepared the clinical room and informed both Shona and her mother what was going to happen. Shona's mother declined the invitation to accompany her into the clinical room but preferred to wait outside. In the clinical room there was Shona, the doctor and Kelsey.

Eventually the cannula was sited and the infusion commenced but Shona was very agitated and distressed as this had required several attempts, five in total. By this time Shona's mother was also very distressed and angry, so much so that she complained to the nurse in charge.

Later that day Kelsey's mentor takes her aside and asks her what happened, specifically why Kelsey did not ask for assistance and why she did not follow the ward guidelines. Kelsey replieds that she was not aware that there were guidelines and that the doctor did not say he wanted to stop. She also says that she could see everyone was busy.

Key questions

Below are a series of questions related to the case study. Read the questions carefully and then write your responses in your professional development portfolio. After this compare your answers with the suggestions on pages 129–132.

1 What are the main issues arising from this case study?

2 What does the context of practice in this case study suggest to you about the learning environment of this placement?
3 Was Kelsey appropriately supervised?
4 How could this situation have been prevented?
5 How could the mentor have used the information from previous placements?
6 What are the legal and ethical implications for the mentor arising from this case study?
7 What different approaches could the mentor and the ward team take to improve the learning environment for students?
8 How can the mentor address the inter-professional working relationship between student nurses and other healthcare professionals?

Possible sources of materials to inform your knowledge and practice

DH (Department of Health) (2004) *The NHS Knowledge and Skills Framework (NHS KSF) and the Development Review Process*. London: DH.

Dimond, B. (2005) *Legal Aspects of Nursing*, 4th edn. Harlow: Longman.

Downie, C.M. and Basford, P. (eds) (2002) *Teaching and Assessing in Clinical Practice*. London: Greenwich University Press.

Gopee, N. (2004) Effective clinical learning in primary care settings, *Nursing Standard*, 18(37): 33–7.

Hand, H. (2006) Promoting effective teaching and learning in the clinical setting, *Nursing Standard*, 20(39): 55–63.

Hendrick, J. (2004) *Law and Ethics*. Cheltenham: Nelson Thornes.

McAllister, L., Lincoln, M., McLeod, S. and Maloney, D. (eds) (1997) *Facilitating Learning in Clinical Settings*. Cheltenham: Nelson Thornes Ltd.

Mideley, K. (2006) Pre-registration student nurses' perception of the hospital learning environment during clinical placements, *Nurse Education Today*, 26: 338–45.

Morris, R. (2004) Speak up or shut up? Accountability and the student nurse, *Paediatric Nursing*, 16(6): 20–22.

NMC (Nursing and Midwifery Council) (2004) *Code of Professional Conduct: Standards for Conduct, Performance and Ethics*. London: NMC.

NMC (2008) *Standards to Support Learning and Assessment in Practice: NMC Standards for Mentors, Practice Teachers and Teachers*. London: NMC.

Quinn, F. (2000) *Principles and Practice of Nurse Education*, 4th edn. Cheltenham: Stanley Thornes Ltd.

Case Study 7

Evidence-based Practice

Before commencing on this case study it is important for you to have reviewed the Nursing and Midwifery Standard for Evidence-based Practice.

This case study offers you the opportunity to explore how evidence-based practice can influence student learning. It can be analysed and reflected upon individually or discussed with peers in a group situation. It specifically relates to the NMC Standard: Evidence-based Practice

The outcomes for this standard are:

- Contribute to strategies to increase or review the evidence base used to support practice.
- Support students in applying an evidence base to their own practice.
- Identify and apply research and **evidence-based practice** to their area of practice.

(NMC 2008a: 21)

This case study has also been mapped to the NHS KSF (DH 2004), which consists of a range of core and specific dimensions that describe the knowledge and skills that mentors will need to apply in their job role. It relates specifically to the following:

Core dimensions 1 to 6

Specific dimensions

- IK1 – Information Processing
- IK2 – Information Collection and Analysis
- IK3 – Knowledge and Information Resources
- G1 – Learning and Development
- G6 – People Management

Case study

Josie is a student nurse on placement at the beginning of the third year of her training. At your initial meeting with her you review the section of her personal development plan where Josie has identified the knowledge and skills that she needs to develop whilst undertaking the placement. Josie has identified that a particular area for development is her knowledge of how research is used to influence patient care.

Prior to her midpoint interview Josie brings two journal articles that she has located to show you. These articles relate to the clinical nursing skills that she needs to develop as part of her placement experience. Josie asks whether the recommendations made in the article should be used to inform the way in which she provides care for the patients in this placement area. As part of the discussion Josie asks how the Trust ensures that policies, guidelines and care pathways are updated as new evidence becomes available.

Towards the end of her placement you are both involved in the care of a patient who is unsure whether the planned nursing intervention is compatible with his personal beliefs. Josie asks how the patient's views and best research evidence can be combined as part of the decision-making process in this case.

Key questions

Below are a series of questions related to the case study. Read the questions carefully and then write your responses in your professional development portfolio. After this compare your answers with the suggestions on pages 132–134.

1 How would you plan to support Josie's learning to facilitate the meeting of the development need identified in her professional development portfolio?
2 How can you encourage Josie to inform herself in relation to evidence-based practice?
3 How would you assess Josie's competency to provide a rationale based on best evidence to justify safe nursing practice?
4 How would you assess Josie's competency at questioning nursing practice in terms of its evidence base?
5 How would you assess Josie's ability to search for new evidence which may have an impact upon patient care?
6 What are the professional and ethical implications for the mentor and the student in relation to this case study?
7 Are there any implications for the Trust, the higher education institution and the public arising out of this case study?

Possible sources of materials to inform your knowledge and practice

Charity site

Mind http://www.mind.org.uk (Accessed 27 February 2010).
This site provides high-quality information and advice, and campaigns to promote and protect good mental health for everyone.

Evidence-based practice web resources

Bandolier http://www.medicine.ox.ac.uk/bandolier/ (Accessed 27 February 2010). Includes all sorts of useful information and considers the evidence for healthcare – in less detail than the Cochrane reviews.

Health Information Resources http://www.library.nhs.uk/default.aspx (Accessed 27 February 2010).
This is an important source of evidence for healthcare and is freely available through the National electronic Library for Health (NeLH). Systematic reviews provide a good idea of the strength of evidence in published research.

Intute Nursing, midwifery and allied professions subject gateway http://www.intute.ac.uk/healthandlifesciences/nursing/ (Accessed 27 February 2010).

National Library of Medicine: Health Services/Technology Assessment Text http://www.ncbi.nlm.nih.gov/books/bv.fcgi?rid=hstat (Accessed 27 February 2010).
This is an American government website which includes links to lots of guidelines e.g. Agency for Healthcare Research and Quality (AHRQ) Evidence-based Clinical Information.

Netting the Evidence http://www.shef.ac.uk/scharr/ir/netting/ (Accessed 27 February 2010).
Provides lots of links to resources about evidence-based healthcare practice.

NHS Scotland Educational Resources Clinical Governance http://www.clinicalgovernance.scot.nhs.uk/ (Accessed 27 February 2010).
This website aims to help you use clinical governance and risk management quality improvement methods in your work. You can use this website in three ways: as a programme of learning, reference source, or training resource.

NurseScribe: Evidence-based nursing (and medicine) http://www.enursescribe.com/evidencebased.htm (Accessed 27 February 2010).
A free database of quality websites selected and evaluated by subject experts. The database is maintained and updated by the higher education community.

Government and statistical sites

Centre for Evidence-based Medicine http://www.cebm.net/ (Accessed 7 July 2007).

Centre for Evidence-based Mental Health Care http://www.cebmh.com/ (Accessed 27 February 2010).

Aims to promote the teaching and practice of evidence-based health care (EBHC) throughout the UK (with special emphasis on evidence-based mental health) and internationally. To develop, evaluate, and disseminate improved methods of using research in practice, and incorporate these in the teaching methods of the CEBMH.

Centre for Reviews and Dissemination, University of York http://www.york.ac.uk/inst/crd/ (Accessed 27 February 2010).
There is a lot of useful information on this site e.g. Database of Abstracts of Reviews of Effects (DARE), publications e.g. *Effective Healthcare* bulletins, lots of links.

Clinical Evidence http://www.clinicalevidence.com/ceweb/conditions/index.jsp (Accessed 27 February 2010).
This BMJ site aims to provide summaries of the evidence for effective health care.

Department for Education and Skills http://www.dfes.gov.uk (Accessed 27 February 2010).

Department of Health http://www.dh.gov.uk (Accessed 27 February 2010).
This site offers policy, guidance and publications for NHS and social care professionals.

National Health Service (NHS) Service Delivery and Organization (SDO) http://www.sdo.lshtm.ac.uk/ (Accessed 27 February 2010).
This is the website for a national research programme set up to develop the evidence base on the organization, management and delivery of healthcare services. Publications available include *Managing Change in Health Care*.

National Institute for Clinical Excellence (NICE) clinical guidelines http://www.nice.org.uk/page.aspx?o=cg (Accessed 27 February 2010).
This is an important site for evidence-based healthcare.

Neighbourhood Statistics http://www.neighbourhood.statistics.gov.uk (Accessed 27 February 2010).
This search allows you to find a **summary report** for your **local neighbourhood**. If you want to know more about the neighbourhood you live or work in, use this search.

North West Public Health Observatory http://www.nwpho.org.uk (Accessed 27 February 2010).
North West Public Health Statistics.

Office for National Statistics (ONS) http://www.statistics.gov.uk (Accessed 27 February 2010).

OMNI http://www.omni.ac.uk/ (Accessed 27 February 2010).
A good source of links to resources in health and medicine.

PRODIGY http://www.cks.nhs.uk/home (Accessed 27 February 2010).
Includes lots of evidence-based information aimed at primary healthcare professionals but also relevant to others.

Public Health Resources Unit sources of evidence http://www.phru.nhs.uk/Pages/PHD/resources.htm (Accessed 16 February 2010).
The Critical Appraisal Skills Programme (CASP) has helped to develop an evidence-based approach in health and social care, working with local, national and international groups.

Scottish Intercollegiate Guidelines Network (SIGN) http://www.sign.ac.uk/guidelines/index.html (Accessed 27 February 2010).
This is a useful site for guidelines for evidence-based healthcare.

UK Government http://www.direct.gov.uk (Accessed 27 February 2010).

Univadis Bandolier articles http://www.msdforphysicians.co.uk/bandolier/bandolierteaser.asp (Accessed 27 February 2010).
Univadis is a website for UK doctors. Some of these Bandolier articles, listed with links, may be useful to you e.g. care pathways, quality and validity of research, the importance of the size of studies.

Journal sources

Evidence-Based Nursing (2005) Purpose and procedure. 8: 66–7. http://www.ebn.bmjjournals.co m/cgi/content/full/8/3/66 (Accessed 27 February 2010).
The general purpose of *Evidence-Based Nursing* is to select from the health-related literature those articles reporting studies and reviews that warrant immediate attention by nurses attempting to keep pace with important advances in their profession.
French, P. (2002) What is the evidence on evidence-based nursing? An epistemological concern, *Journal of Advanced Nursing*, 37(3): 250–57.
Kitson, A. (2002) Recognising relationships: reflections on evidence-based practice, *Nursing Inquiry*, 9(3): 179–94.
Rycroft-Malone, J., Seers, K., Titchen, A., Harvey, G., Kitson, A. and McCormack, B. (2004) What counts as evidence in evidence-based practice?, *Journal of Advanced Nursing*, 47(1): 81–90.

NHS sites

Guidelines finder http://www.library.nhs.uk/guidelinesfinder/AboutUs.aspx (Accessed 27 February 2010).
UK approved evidence-based clinical guidelines available on the internet in full text.

Protocols and Care Pathways specialist library http://www.library.nhs.uk/pathways/ (Accessed 27 February 2010).
For health professionals who are developing, implementing and evaluating care pathways and clinical protocols.

Qualitative appraisal tools

Appraisal tools available on the web which are specifically designed for qualitative research include:
Qualitative research in health care: three articles from the *British Medical Journal*: Assessing quality in qualitative research http://www.bmj.bmjjournals.com/cgi/content/full/320/7226/50 (Accessed 27 February 2010).
Analysing qualitative data http://www.bmj.bmjjournals.com/cgi/content/full/320/7227/114 (Accessed 27 February 2010).
Using qualitative methods in health related action research http://www.bmj.bmjjournals.com/cgi/content/full/320/7228/178 (Accessed 27 February 2010).

Case Study 8

Leadership

Before commencing on this case study it is important for you to have reviewed the Nursing and Midwifery Standard for Leadership

This case study offers you the opportunity to explore the leadership responsibilities of the mentor. It can be analysed and reflected upon individually or discussed with peers in a group situation. It specifically relates to the NMC Standard: Leadership.

The outcomes for this standard are:

- Plan a series of learning experiences that will meet students' defined learning needs.
- Be an advocate for students by supporting them in accessing learning opportunities that meet their individual needs – involving a range of other professionals, patients, clients and carers.
- Prioritize work to accommodate support of students within their practice roles.
- Provide feedback about the effectiveness of learning and assessment in practice.

(NMC 2008: 21)

This case study has also been mapped to the NHS KSF (DH 2004), which consists of a range of core and specific dimensions that describe the knowledge and skills that mentors will need to apply in their job role. It relates specifically to the following:

Core dimensions 1 to 6

Specific dimensions

- IK1 – Information Processing
- IK2 – Information Collection and Analysis
- IK3 – Knowledge and Information Resources

- G1 – Learning and Development
- G6 – People Management.

Case study

Braxton Ward is a continuing care area for *(select the branch which is appropriate to you)*. There have been students placed here successfully for at least 10 years although recently there have been several staff changes. Only one of the four senior staff remains in post. All of the junior staff have been in their positions for over seven years. The new manager, George Hicks, has two experienced but new (Band 6) senior staff and a staff member, Vivian Cheynes, who was recently unsuccessful in applying for George's post.

The two new senior staff (Albert Stokes and John Brompton) were asking to undertake the degree-level mentorship module but George has never been able to find the time to organize their development or the resources to fund it. George's time is often taken up in settling disputes between the established junior members of staff, which he does fairly but repeatedly.

Vivian is already a mentor and has taken on a newly placed student who must undertake a four-week period of remedial practice, having failed his previous summative assessment. George, who is a qualified mentor, is happy to have Vivian undertake the supervision as the complexities of remedial supervision currently have a lower priority than clinical work. George receives an unexpected letter from Vivian informing him that she has been successful in obtaining a promotion. Vivian does not return to duty but provides a sick note for four weeks.

The student is subsequently supervised by Albert Stokes; however, there has been no liaison beforehand between him and Vivian. After the four-week placement the student comes to George with his documentation, which George refuses to sign as he has not worked with him.

George receives a phone call from a concerned personal teacher.

Key questions

Below are a series of questions related to the case study. Read the questions carefully and then write your responses in your professional development portfolio. After this compare your answers with the suggestions on pages 134–137.

1 At what level does leadership take place in an organization and specifically

on Braxton ward? Using the leadership standards of the NMC as guidelines, identify whether leadership has failed in this instance?
2   What are the major elements of leadership and how does this link to the role of the practice placement manager and mentor in this case study?
3   Who, in this case study, was and wasn't exercising leadership in relation to this student?
4   What do you think George's priorities should have been?
5   What actions should be undertaken at the organizational and individual level to address this case study?

Possible sources of materials to inform your knowledge and practice

Broome, A. (1997) *Managing Change (Essentials of Nursing Management)*. Basingstoke: Palgrave Macmillan.

Buchanan, D. and Huczynski, A. (2001) *Organisational Behaviour: An Introductory Text*, 4th edn. London: Prentice Hall.

Clarke, J. and Copcutt, L. (1997) *Management for Nurses and Healthcare Professionals*. Edinburgh: Churchill Livingstone.

Cole, G.A. (2000) *Management Theory and Practice*, 5th edn. London: Continuum.

DH (Department of Health) (2004) *The NHS Knowledge and Skills Framework (NHS KSF) and the Development Review Process*. London: DH.

Girvin, J. (1998) *Leadership in Nursing (Essentials of Nursing Management)*. Basingstoke: Palgrave Macmillan.

Iles, V. (2006) *Really Managing Healthcare*, 2nd edn. Maidenhead: Open University Press.

Kermally, S. (1999) *The Management Tool Kit*. London: Thorogood.

Marquis, B. and Huston, C. (1998) *Management Decision Making for Nurses*, 4th edn. Philadelphia, PA: Lippincott.

Marriner-Tomey, A. (2000) *Nursing Management and Leadership*, 5th edn. New York: Mosby.

Moullin, M. (2002) *Delivering Excellence in Health and Social Care*. Maidenhead: Open University Press.

Mullins, L. (2007) *Management and Organisational Behaviour*, 8th edn. Harlow: Prentice Hall.

NMC (Nursing and Midwifery Council) (2008) *Standards to Support Learning and Assessment in Practice: NMC Standards for Mentors, Practice Teachers and Teachers*. London: NMC.

Rocchiccioli, J. and Tilbury, M. (1998) *Clinical Leadership in Nursing*. London: Saunders.

Sullivan, E. and Decker, P. (2001) *Effective Leadership and Management in Nursing*, 5th edn. London: Prentice Hall.

Thompson, N. (2002) *People Skills*, 2nd edn. Basingstoke: Palgrave Macmillan.

Wadderburn Tate, C. (1999) *Leadership in Nursing*. Edinburgh: Churchill Livingstone.

Journals

Clinical Governance: An International Journal
Health Service Journal
International Journal of Healthcare Quality Assurance
Journal of Nursing Management

Websites

Department of Health http://www.DH.gov.uk (Accessed 17 February 2010).
National Health Service http://www.nhs.uk (Accessed 17 February 2010).
Institute of Healthcare Management http://www.ihm.org.uk/professional-development-learning (Accessed 17 February 2010).

Case Study 9

Group Assessment Exercise

We will complete this section of the book by asking you to undertake an assessment exercise within a group because to be maintained on the local **live register** of mentors, the NMC Standards (2008:12) state that you should have:

> Explored as a group activity the validity and reliability of judgements made when assessing practice in challenging circumstances. The completion of the following exercise will enable you to provide evidence that you have done this.

You can meet this requirement by undertaking the following exercise:

Assessment exercise case study

A second-year student has reached the final week of her placement. As the mentor you discover that the student has difficulty in completing written records of care. This problem only came to light when she was asked to complete a care plan under your supervision. The student informs you that she is dyslexic but does not tell anyone, to avoid being stereotyped. Discuss the following questions with your peers on your placement.

Below are a series of questions related to the case study. Read the questions carefully and then discuss your responses as a group. Once you have done this, compare your answers to those suggested in the Appendix. You may find that you wish to expand your own responses after reading these.

Key questions

Below are a series of questions related to the case study.

We would recommend that you read the questions carefully and then discuss your different viewpoints as a group. Nominate somebody within the group to take notes and to summarize at the end of your discussion. Once you have done this, write your own responses in your professional development portfolio. The purpose of this exercise is to appreciate the varying opinions which can then be compared to the suggestions on pages 138–139.

1 As a group, identify the key issues arising from this case study.
2 Agree what actions the mentor should take.
3 Identify any practice placement resources which would help the mentor in this situation.
4 As a group, establish what you think are the needs of the student here.
5 What are the professional responsibilities for the mentor in this situation?

Summary

This section of the book has provided you with a flexible, self-directed alternative to your updating and continuing development as a mentor using a case study approach. Examples from practice have been used which mimic real situations that could happen to you in your practice setting.

By completing the case studies you have engaged in problem solving, analysis, reflection and evaluation in order to develop your knowledge and future practice related to the associated standard.

Key points

- Two or three mentorship standards should be completed over a 12-month period.
- All eight mentorship standards must be completed over a three-year period.
- A group assessment exercise must also be completed to meet the NMC Standards (2008b).
- Evidence generated from the activities should demonstrate how you have maintained your ongoing knowledge and competence as a practising mentor within your practice area.
- Evidence can be assembled in your professional development portfolio and demonstrated to your reviewer at your annual appraisal.

Before you move on to the next chapter, start to consider other activities and types of evidence which could complement those that you have identified from completing this chapter.

These could then be useful to you when you when you providing evidence of how you are maintaining your ongoing competence and also to support your mentorship development/updating.

Part 3

Updating and Sources of Evidence

5

Mentor Updating: Other Activities/Sources of Evidence

Cyril Murray and Lyn Rosen

Aim

The aim of this chapter is to outline activities and types of evidence which can be applied to maintain your ongoing competence.

Learning outcomes

After reading this chapter you will be able to:

- identify activities which link to your appraisal and personal development plans that could be undertaken on an annual basis to support your mentorship development/updating;
- identify sources of evidence which could be presented to demonstrate your ongoing competence.

The Nursing and Midwifery Council regulations

The previous section in the book enabled you, by using a case study approach, to understand the link between the eight mandatory standards (NMC 2008a) and the Knowledge and Skills Framework (DH 2004) in order to promote, maintain and record your own ongoing competence.

This chapter offers other approaches you could use to develop and maintain your ongoing competence as a mentor. Through a range of short activities you will explore the links between your appraisal and personal development plans and the demonstration of your ongoing competence as a mentor.

Before considering this, it is important to remind you of the specific Nursing and Midwifery Council (NMC) regulatory codes you must comply with as part of your professional role that relate to teaching and learning in practice.

- First, the Nursing and Midwifery Council (NMC) requires you as a registrant, through its Code of Professional Conduct (NMC 2008b: 7), to 'keep your knowledge and skills up to date throughout your working life and . . . have the knowledge and skills for safe and effective practice'. This is very important as a mentor as you will be expected to facilitate, supervise and assess students' learning and performance.
- Secondly, the NMC Code (NMC 2008b: 5) states: 'You must facilitate students and others to develop their competence'. Again as a mentor you will be expected to do this whenever you work with students. The development of students' knowledge, skills and attitudes for safe and effective practice needs mentors who are committed to the teaching and learning process (Benner 1984).
- In addition the NMC requires you as a mentor to attend an update on a regular basis. 'Regular' is interpreted as annual and the *Standards to Support Learning and Assessment in Practice* (NMC 2008a) actually stipulate this. Practitioners who are mentors are required to demonstrate how they have maintained their knowledge and competence in relation to the standards above (NMC 2008a).
- Finally, the Post-registration Education and Practice (PREP) guidelines (NMC 2005) require all practitioners to fulfil the continuing professional development (CPD) standard for re-registration purposes. This includes a commitment to undertake continuing professional development (CPD) of at least 35 hours of learning activity relevant to your practice during the three years prior to your renewal of registration relevant to your practice, and to maintain a personal professional portfolio of this learning activity.

Identify activities which link to the appraisal and personal development planning processes to support mentorship development/updating

In Chapter 2 a description was offered on how your ongoing competence as a mentor could be linked to your annual employer-led appraisal, and your triennial review of mentor competency (NMC 2008a). The following activities could help you meet both your professional and employer requirements.

Activity 5.1

Read carefully your post outline (DH 2004). This will enable you to understand the contractual and professional responsibilities relating to to your role. Take into consideration the definition of mentorship presented in Chapter 1 on page 6.

From looking at your post outline can you tease out the stated requirements that are needed for you to fulfil the role of a mentor? Whilst the word mentor or mentorship may not be present there will be descriptors that implicitly identify what you are required to do within your role and in respect of maintaining your knowledge and skills.

Whilst a post outline differs for each role you have, you may have picked up some of the following terms in yours which can be related to your role as a mentor:

- communicate with others;
- contribute to service improvements;
- enhance the quality of care;
- promote equality and diversity;
- promote the health and well-being of others;
- enable people to learn and develop;
- plan, co-ordinate, facilitate, supervise and assess the work of others.

Activity 5.2

Access the following links

1 http://www.dh.gov.uk/prod_consum_dh/groups/dh_digitalassets/@dh/@en/documents/digitalasset/dh_4105481.pdf
   This link provides an example of a full NHS KSF outline for a post (DH 2004). Whilst the post is for a Post Grade Occupational Therapist the principles can be transferred to nursing.

2 Section 2.1.2 pages 20 and 21 of the NMC *Standards to Support Learning and Assessment in Practice* (NMC 2008a) at http://www.nmc-uk.org/aDisplayDocument.aspx?documentID=4368

These domains and outcomes can provide the framework for assessing, developing and demonstrating your ongoing competence as a mentor.

3 The NMC Code: *Standards of Conduct, Performance and Ethics for Nurses and Midwives* (NMC 2008b) at http://www.nmc-uk.org/aArticle.aspx?ArticleID=3056

This will clarify your professional obligations to the profession, specifically in relation to your educational sub-role.

Analyse these documents and then review your post outline again. Identify the areas of application which apply to your mentor role.

Carefully read the Table 5.1, as it offers you an example of how the NHS KSF, the NMC standards and NMC Code could be reviewed to identify areas of application specific to the role of a mentor.

You may have found the process time-consuming and challenging but once you have completed Activity 5.2 you will have a clearer idea of what is expected from you in your role as a mentor, the associated professional body and the contractual obligations that are identified in your post outline. The activity will also help you to identify any areas for further development which you can discuss with your appraiser/reviewer at your personal development planning meeting as part of your annual appraisal/triennial review.

Activity 5.3

Having completed the two previous activities, start to record in your professional development portfolio any areas for further development that you have identified.

This will help you at your next appraisal as you will have prepared work in readiness for discussion.

Table 5.1 An example of how the NHS KSF, the NMC Standards and NMC Code could be reviewed to identify areas of application specific to the role of a mentor

Source of information	Core components	Possible example areas of application to your role as a mentor
NHS KSF (DH 2004) post outline Dimension: Service Improvement Level 2: Contribution to the implementation of services	*Indicators* 1 Discuss and agree with the work team: • the implications of direction, policies and strategies on your current practice; • the changes that they can make as a team; • the changes you can make as an individual; • how to take the changes forward. 2 Constructively makes agreed changes to one's own work in the agreed timescale seeking support as and when necessary. 3 Support others in understanding the need for and making agreed changes. 4 Evaluate one's own and others' work when required to do so, completing the relevant documentation. 5 Make constructive suggestions as to how services can be improved for users and the public. 6 Constructively identify issues with direction, policies and strategies in the interests of users and the public.	1 Carry out student/staff interviews (reviewing and refining one's performance) which evaluate their learning and assessment experiences in the placement. 2 Become actively involved with the practice education lead (PEL) on each placement, other mentors and the university link teacher in placement audits and student evaluations of the learning environment and the action plans arising from both of these activities. 3 Organize team meetings to discuss student learning and assessment experiences, the professional body, Trust and/or university policies relating to education and practice and the changes needed to implement these e.g. maintaining an ongoing record of student achievement. 4 Set up systems/processes for identifying and discussing empirical evidence to inform one's own and others' nursing practices e.g. research boards, local journal club, teaching and learning packs. 5 Develop resources which enable evidence to become available for reviewing and appraising current practices e.g. electronic sources, journals etc.
NMC *Standards to Support Learning and Assessment in Practice* (NMC 2008)	**Domain 4 Evaluation of learning** **Outcome** *Contribute to the evaluation of student learning and assessment experiences – proposing aspects for change resulting from such evaluation.* **Domain 5 Creating an environment for learning** **Outcome** *Identify aspects of the learning environment which could be enhanced – negotiating with others to make appropriate changes.*	6 Review and develop the learning resources with other team members e.g. identification and selection of teaching/learning packs, spoke placements, staff profile of expertise/learning opportunities in placement, electronic resources on placement. *(Continued Overleaf)*

Table 5.1 Continued

Source of information	Core components	Possible example areas of application to your role as a mentor
	Domain 6 Context of practice	7 Develop structured plans which link learning opportunities within the learning environment to students' objectives e.g. pre-registration proficiencies, and monitor their effectiveness.
	Outcomes Contribute to the development of an environment in which effective practice is fostered, implemented, evaluated and disseminated.	
	Set and maintain professional boundaries that are sufficiently flexible for providing interprofessional care.	8 Promote the development of team mentorship/ preceptorship activities.
	Initiate and respond to practice developments to ensure safe and effective care is achieved and an effective learning environment is maintained.	9 Attend events which provide information on mentoring, supporting learners and development of effective learning environments and educational or practice policy changes.
	Domain 7 Evidence-based practice	10 Read, reflect and/or apply knowledge via formal updating study days or informal work-based learning/self-directed learning in relation to:
	Outcomes Identify and apply research and evidence-based practice to your area of practice.	• educational evaluation – student, self or peer; • facilitation of learning; • assessment;
	Contribute to strategies to increase or review the evidence base used to support practice.	• change management; • quality/service development; • coaching others; • role modelling; • types of evidence; • appraising research; • implementation and dissemination of research findings;
	Some key statements	• risk management; • promoting an inter-professional care service; • team working; • promotion of reflective practice.
NMC *Standards of Conduct, Performance and Ethics for Nurses and Midwives* (NMC 2008)	1 The people in your care must be able to trust you with their health and well-being. To justify that trust you must: • make the care of people your first concern, treating them as individuals and respecting their dignity; • work with others to protect and promote the health and well-being of those in your care; • provide a high standard of practice at all times.	11 Identify and utilize tools for self and/or peer evaluation.
	2 As a professional you are personally accountable for actions or omissions in your practice and must always be able to justify your decisions.	
	3 You must deliver care based upon the best available evidence or best practice.	

The appraisal (development review process)/personal development planning

Normally an appraisal or development review process is an ongoing cycle involving a review of an individual's performance against the criteria of their post outline. The NHS KSF (DH 2004) identified the following four stages associated with this process:

1 A joint review of the staff member's work against the post outline.
2 The development of a personal development plan.
3 Learning and development activities undertaken by the staff member supported by the appraiser/reviewer.
4 An evaluation of the learning and development which has occurred and application of this in practice.

To prepare for the joint review you need to review your post outline undertaken in Activity 5.1 and consider your work in detail against this.

Remember that the requirement of being a mentor and maintaining your ongoing competence for this role is one part of your overall review against the demands of your post.

Your personal development plan may look something like Table 5.2.

Table 5.2 An example of a personal development plan

What is the developmental need?	What will I do to develop myself?	How will I know I have done this?	What is the planned date for completion?	What support do I need and where will I get it from?	What are the barriers and how can I overcome these?
To become a sign-off mentor and be recognized on the live register in relation to this professional role.	Identify a sign-off mentor to supervise and assess my practice. Contact the university link teacher for advice on issues associated with this role. Liaise with other sign-off mentors on the problems, pitfalls and good practices associated with this role. Discuss with them the issues of accountability associated with decisions for passing or failing students when assessing their proficiency levels at the end of a programme.	Been supervised on three separate occasions by an existing sign-off mentor. Been signed off as competent to become a sign-off mentor and recorded as such on the live register. Possess confidence and understanding of the responsibilities and accountability associated with this important professional role	To be agreed. Within the next 12 months.	I need support from other sign-off mentors, the university link teacher and my appraiser/reviewer. Time built into my daily work role to undertake and achieve the requirements to become a sign-off mentor. This includes time for discussions with others, literature searching and reviewing evidence in the Trust library on the subject and supervision and assessment time with a sign-off mentor on the placement.	Time built into the daily work routine for me and my sign-off mentor. This needs to be facilitated by the placement manager and the appraiser/reviewer in discussion with myself.

SWOT analysis

A useful tool to help you identify your personal development needs is known as a SWOT analysis (Mullins 1996). SWOT refers to:

- strengths;
- weaknesses;
- opportunities;
- threats.

In other words, once you have identified the areas within your job role related to your mentor role, think about what you are good at (strengths) and not so good at (weaknesses). Strengths and weaknesses are considered to be internal factors affecting your performance in a particular role, so really are about *you*.

Opportunities and threats relate to the external factors affecting your performance as a mentor, so take time to think about issues related to your practice area which might impact on how well you do your job as a mentor.

When completing your SWOT analysis it is important not just to come up with a list of strengths and weaknesses but also to consider how you can improve on these.

From this you can then discuss your development needs and create a learning and development plan with your reviewer/appraiser on how these areas of weakness can be addressed so that your ongoing competence as a mentor can be met.

Example

You have completed nine months' experience as a qualified mentor. During this time you have carried out a couple of student assessments but now need to understand and fulfil the requirements in becoming a sign-off mentor as there are not enough of these on your ward.

Your SWOT analysis could look like this:

Strengths

- I have undertaken a number of student assessments on the placement area.
- I have provided constructive feedback to students and assisted them in identifying future learning needs and actions.
- I have managed and supported failing students.
- I understand the curriculum and assessment process and have a sound knowledge of the different assessment strategies used.

- I participate with other mentors on the placement in discussing and providing evidence about student/staff performance.
- I am aware of my professional responsibilities as a mentor and as a nurse.
- I am aware of NMC criteria to become a sign-off mentor (NMC 2008a, NMC 2010)

Weaknesses

- I am unable to assess students on their final assessment of practice as I am not qualified as a sign-off mentor.
- I need to develop an in-depth understanding of the issues of accountability associated with decisions for passing or failing students when assessing their proficiency levels at the end of a programme.

Opportunities

- There are students who are undertaking a final placement and who require an assessment of their proficiency levels for entry to the professional register.
- There are existing sign-off mentors on placement who can supervise, support and assess my abilities in becoming a sign-off mentor.
- There are excellent relationships with higher education and support from the university link teacher.

Threats

- Time constraint pressures to existing sign-off mentors to supervise, support and assess my abilities.

Identify evidence for ongoing competence

During the evaluation stage of your developmental review you will have to present evidence on the effectiveness of the developmental plan in relation to enhancing your knowledge and skills for your post, the application of this in practice and the demonstration of your ongoing competence as a mentor.

The nature and type of evidence can take many forms, for example:

- direct observation by the appraiser/reviewer of your actual performance in practice;
- discussions similar to a viva voce which demonstrate underpinning knowledge;
- media and IT items such as videos, CDs, or even paper-based information.

There are no limits to this so try to be creative and produce a wide range of evidence to discuss with your appraiser/reviewer. By doing this you may find that some evidence can be used to demonstrate competence against a number of developmental activities.

Activity 5.4

With regard to the example above about the developmental plan to become a sign-off mentor, can you think about what evidence could be submitted to your appraiser/reviewer to demonstrate that you had achieved this?

The following types of evidence could have been considered:

- Discussions with your appraiser/reviewer about how you have applied the knowledge and skills gained in practice and your in-depth understanding of the responsibilities associated with signing off student proficiency for entry to the professional register.
- A written testimony from your sign-off mentor that you are competent to fulfil this professional role.
- Photocopied documentation that you have completed three final student assessments (anonymized) and relevant Trust documentation verifying that you have met the requirements to become a sign-off mentor.
- A photocopy of your entry onto the live register as a sign-off mentor.
- Testimonies from others such as existing mentors or university staff on issues related to student assessments.

What other sources of evidence can I use?

Throughout this book we have emphasized the importance of reviewing and maintaining your competence against the eight domains and learning outcomes of the NMC standards for mentors (NMC 2008). You should complete the above activities to help you identify your current abilities and developmental needs in line with your appraisal/developmental review.

One key element that you will have to consider is the different types of evidence to present that demonstrate that you have acquired the knowledge and skills associated with your post. There are many different sources of evidence that you may be able to collect and present.

The focus should be on originality, creativity and providing the best examples of how the criteria of the mandatory standards have been achieved.

The list below offers examples of different types of evidence that might be presented. It is by no means an exhaustive list, but should be used to generate ideas of other examples.

Articles from journals

It may be useful to include articles from journals as a way of complementing the reading that you have undertaken. However, the article needs to be accompanied by either a reflective commentary in relation to the contents provided in the article or how you have used the information in your work. A regurgitation of the contents of the article is not appropriate. You could also discuss the contents as a way of demonstrating your underpinning knowledge and application in practice.

Assessment documents from students

Any assessment documents which are provided should have the student's name removed but should be photocopies of the original papers. It is useful to include the assessment documentation and any personal development plans with a short summary of what occurred in the event e.g. how you provided feedback to the student.

Audits/action plans

You may include the audit and relevant action plan from your area as evidence but, again, it would be useful to include how you have used the information in your area of work. For example, the learning resources may have been identified as an area requiring action and it may be possible for you to have started to develop a system for providing some new aids within your area of work. Student evaluations of the learning environment or the audit by the University of the Learning Environment could lead to the development of action plans which you might engage in but they must show your specific input.

Course development

You may include any documentary evidence about your contribution to course development e.g. feedback from the university link teacher, **placement educational lead**, or Course Development Team.

Educational updates

You may have participated in an educational update meeting between the placement educational leads and a member from the university who covers your ward/Trust. A record may be kept of the meeting and any subsequent actions which you agreed to undertake. This could be complemented by other documentary evidence in terms of your involvement following the educational update e.g. verification letters.

Evaluations

You may undertake an evaluation of a professional/government document related to nurse education and summarize its implications in practice.

Induction/orientation packs

These may be developed by you. If you choose to do so, it might be useful to produce an outline document and circulate it to the other team members for their comments before developing it. Otherwise the actual induction or orientation pack can be submitted.

Information notice boards

For example, you could use this medium to showcase information related to evidence-based practice initiatives. Photographs of the display board chronicled in your portfolio could be used as a basis for discussion at your review.

Learning log

A learning log may be completed in order to encapsulate a significant event for you in respect of an educational issue.

Learning packages

You could develop these, but you would be strongly advised not to do so, as they are very time-consuming documents. Other sources of information to promote learning are generally more effective e.g. articles on a research board etc.

Literature review

You may include a synopsis of this in relation to a particular topic area.

Minutes of meetings

The same principles apply to this as to the report section below. These could be with other mentors, the placement educational leads or university representatives about educational/practice policies, changes etc. Your specific input/output needs to be transparent.

RCN student toolkit

This may be used in order to assess how effective the mentorship support and learning environment for students is. This toolkit could be used in conjunction with the nursing audit documentation or other evidence which you have gleaned in respect of assessing and improving the learning environment in which you work.

Reflective commentaries

Any reflective processes which are utilized should demonstrate the inclusion of a reflective model. Reflective commentaries should demonstrate your analytical behaviour.

Reports

You may have written a report in relation to a particular aspect of work that you have been involved in. The report should be complemented by any relevant action plan, testimonial etc. in order to show you were involved in writing the report and what the outcomes have been since its production.

Quality of care initiatives introduced

If you have been involved in any new initiatives you could monitor the adoption, achievement and demonstration of best practice related to these.

Self and peer evaluation activities

You could evaluate your own and others' teaching and learning activities, highlighting good practice and suggesting areas of improvement.

SWOT analysis

SWOT analysis is useful to identify any strengths, weaknesses, opportunities and threats in relation to a particular issue. However, what really needs to accompany the SWOT analysis is some further evidence of how you have used this information through an action plan, a testimonial or a reflective commentary.

Teaching plan

This may be included as part of one or more teaching sessions that you have undertaken in your area of work. It may be useful to include any sort of evaluatory comments that the recipients of the teaching felt.

Testimonials

Testimonials could be obtained from managers, peers, students or significant others. The focus in any testimonial should be upon what you did, why the actions were needed and what the outcomes were. The testimonials should be signed by the relevant person who is providing the information.

Viva voce (oral assessment)

This might enable you to demonstrate underpinning knowledge, linked to goals set at your previous appraisal. This could be particularly effective when linked to a gateway appraisal.

Summary

The aim of this chapter was to outline activities and types of evidence which can be applied to maintain your ongoing competence.

Key points

- The NMC have specific regulatory codes you must comply with as part of your professional role as a mentor.
- Your post outline will identify your contractual (employment) responsibilities as a mentor.
- Each mentor will have a triennial review with their appraiser in relation to their ongoing competence as a mentor.
- A SWOT analysis using your post outline can help you identify your personal development needs and future opportunities as a mentor.
- Examples of evidence to demonstrate your ongoing competence as a mentor were presented as this will be a requirement at a triennial review meeting.

References

Benner, P. (1984) *From Novice to Expert: Excellence and Power in Clinical Nursing Practice.* London: Prentice Hall.

DH (Department of Health) (2004) *The NHS Knowledge and Skills Framework (NHS KSF) and Development Review Process.* London: Department of Health.

Mullins, L. (1996) *Management and Organisational Behaviour*, 4th edn. London: Pitman.

Nursing and Midwifery Council (2005) *The PREP Handbook.* London: NMC.

Nursing and Midwifery Council (2008a) *Standards to Support Learning and Assessment in Practice. NMC Standards for Mentors, Practice Teachers and Teachers.* http://www.nmc-uk.org/aDisplayDocument.aspx?documentID=4368 (Accessed 10 July 2009).

Nursing and Midwifery Council (2008b) *The Code: Standards of Conduct, Performance and Ethics for Nurses and Midwives.* http://www.nmc-uk.org/aArticle.aspx?ArticleID=3056 (Accessed 10 July 2009).

Nursing and Midwifery Council (2010) *Sign Off Mentor Criteria.* NMC Circular 05/2010. Issued 26 March 2010. London: NMC.

6

Conclusion

This book has provided detailed information on how you, as a mentor, can maintain and update your ongoing competence. Before you close the book it might be useful to take a few moments to read two reports, the *Next Stage Review* report (Darzi 2008), which points out that nurses will always be at the heart of shaping patient experience and delivering care, together with the DH (2006) report on *Modernising Nursing Careers: Setting the Direction*. This second document outlines a rapidly changing healthcare arena and identifies the need to respond appropriately as nurses are now expected to undertake many new activities such as setting up new services, working across boundaries and taking on new responsibilities and roles.

Within this context it was logical to review pre-registration nurse training to enable nurses of the future to meet the needs of patients and clients safely and effectively. The recent *Review of Pre-Registration Nursing Education Project: Key Changes to Nursing Education Programmes Following Phase 1* has resulted in the decision to move to an all-graduate nursing profession and the NMC (2009) summarizes the key changes to nursing education programmes as follows:

The minimum award for a nursing qualification will be degree. The common foundation programme and branch model will be replaced by:

- modernised pathways that will lead to registration in one of the four fields of adult, child learning, disability and mental health
- generic and field specific learning throughout the programme
- flexible boundaries between the generic and field specific components with field component increasing over time
- wide opportunities for shared learning

There will be:

- progression points with NMC outcome measures that include community and public health

- an increase in the proportion of practice learning experience to be gained in the community and other environments
- an increase in the maximum proportion of accreditation of prior (experiential) learning (AP(E)L) that can be applied from the current one-third to one-half of the programme.

http://www.nmc-uk.org/aArticle.aspx?ArticleID=3974

Phase 2 of this consultation, which is to take place between January 2009 and August 2010, looks at the knowledge, skills and attitudes that nurses need to provide safe and effective care to their patients and clients.

With these documents in mind you will need to think about what the move to an all-graduate profession will mean for the workforce, service delivery, quality of care and, *more specifically, to you as a mentor.* You may consider whether this move merely brings nursing into line with other healthcare professions and should not affect how nurses work, or whether it is an opportunity to look at the overall shape and scope of the nursing workforce and to develop it in line with future changes in requirements in the delivery of healthcare. Whatever view you take, as a mentor you play a *vital* part in the supervision and assessment of future nurses. It is therefore your responsibility to keep up to date and assess fairly and appropriately within the specified guidelines which are set out in this book. Some key points are set out below, but you should be able to think of many more.

Key points

- You are accountable to the NMC and your employer in relation to your mentoring role and professional updating/competence.
- There will be the need for mentors who are knowledgeable doers to continue promoting quality placements and facilitating inter-professional learning.
- There will be a need for you to identify what the differences are between diploma and graduate learning and assessment in your role as a mentor.
- Mentors now and in the future will need to be up to date and able to demonstrate their ongoing competence to respond to this agenda (i.e. an all-graduate profession).
- There is a need to support the NMC's role in public protection, mentor competence and the maintenance of the live professional register.

We really hope that you have enjoyed this book and that it will help you with the responsibilities of mentoring and your own professional development.

References

Darzi, A. (2008) *High Quality Care for All: NHS Next Stage Review Final Report.* http://www.dh.gov.uk/en/publicationsandstatistics/publications/publicationspolicyandguidance/DH_085825 (Accessed 7 December 2009).

DH (Department of Health) (2006) *Modernising Nursing Careers: Setting the Direction.* http://www.dh.gov.uk/prod_consum_dh/groups/dh_digitalassets/@dh/@en/documents/ digitalasset/dh_4138757.pdf (Accessed 7 December 2009).

NMC (Nursing and Midwifery Council) (2009) *Key Changes to Nurse Education Programmes Following Phase 1.* http://www.nmc-uk.org/aArticle.aspx?ArticleID=3974 (Accessed 7 December 2009).

Appendix

Suggested Answers to the Case Studies

Case Study 1
Standard: Establishing Effective Working Relationships

1 What are the main issues arising from this case study?

The mentor should ascertain what Dawn needs to know in respect of developing relationships and agree it with her. The mentor needs to help Dawn to do the following:

- Outline the types of confidential and sensitive issues that may need special attention.
- Identify the multi-professional and other agencies involved and give an explanation of their role in this context.
- Determine who she needs to develop a working relationship with. Establish whether these are internal or external agencies.
- Initiate contact with multi-professional and other agencies and together discuss how that contact is then maintained and monitored.
- Provide a clear explanation of her own role and responsibilities in this instance (and that of the chair for the meeting).
- Appreciate the importance of presenting and maintaining a professional image of her organization together with an effective working relationship.
- Identify how effective communication forms a part of professional and ethical best practice because nurses have to interact not only with patients and clients but also with a multi-professional and multicultural team to

maximize the quality of care/interventions and minimize any harm to the patients.

2   How are effective working relationships maintained?

- By applying the codes of practice relevant to your professional practice.
- By knowing the importance of effective team work.
- By knowing what 'good working relationships' within the multi-professional team actually means in practice.
- By knowing how to establish good working relationships with the multi-professional team.
- By communicating clearly with the team.
- By undertaking the duties for which you are responsible.
- By participating in team discussions and listening to the suggestions of team members.
- By understanding the procedures for dealing with conflict.
- By understanding the importance of treating individuals equitably.
- By knowing the limits of your authority.
- By knowing the types of situations in which you may need to consult other people for advice and information.
- By knowing how to present yourself and your organization in a positive light.
- By understanding the types of confidential and sensitive issues that may need special attention.

3   What do you have to do to facilitate Dawn's learning in relation to establishing working relationships?

- The role of the mentor in this instance is to discuss and work with the mentee in order to support their learning. You will need to identify what Dawn already knows and plan accordingly. We suggest a useful way to start this might be to ask why a healthcare professional needs to maintain and develop effective working relationships. For instance, you could ask her to list components of both good and poor working relationships.
- You might be in a position to arrange for Dawn to visit various members of the multi-professional team so that she can appreciate their roles. Dawn should also be clear on:
  - ➤ the importance of effective team work;
  - ➤ what 'good working relationships' means in practice;
  - ➤ how to establish good working relationships with members of the multi-professional team;
  - ➤ why it is important to communicate clearly with the multi-professional team;
  - ➤ how to communicate with the team;

- ➤ the duties that she would be responsible for as a qualified member of staff;
- ➤ why it is important to carry out her duties as agreed;
- ➤ situations in which she may need help in her role and duties and why she should always ask for help and information in these situations;
- ➤ situations in which she may need to provide help and information to her co-officials and support staff;
- ➤ why team discussions are important and why she should contribute to them;
- ➤ procedures for dealing with conflict;
- ➤ why it is important to discuss her suggestions with colleagues and to take account of their ideas;
- ➤ why effective communication is important and the most effective way to communicate;
- ➤ when it is important to listen;
- ➤ the importance of treating individuals equitably.

4 What would Dawn's involvement entail?

- You might ask Dawn to contact specific agencies to invite them to the meeting.
- You might ask her to draw up her own ideas for an agenda for the meeting.
- If Dawn is a confident person, she may be happy to be given a role within this first meeting, although it would be quite acceptable for her to observe at this stage, before taking an active role at another meeting before leaving the ward.
- She may wish to be considered the patient's advocate at the meeting. This all needs to be discussed with Dawn.

5 What boundaries, if any, need to be in place?

- Dawn must not feel threatened by being given any responsibility she is not ready for, but should be guided towards this in a constructive way.
- Clear explanations should be offered for actions taken and for decisions that are made.
- If opportunities can be given to meet or work with members of the multi-professional team beforehand, they should be offered.
- It must be clearly established when Dawn should ask for help.

6 What might be the barriers to effective inter-professional working?

Barriers to effective working relationships may involve:

- the team;
- dealing with conflict;

- keeping people informed;
- valuing differences between individuals.

7 What strategies could Dawn utilize to overcome these barriers?

You may wish to ask her to think about how effective her working relationships had been in the past, how they are at present and what might be done to improve them in the future.

8 What is her professional responsibility?

- Refer her to the principles identified within *The Code: Standards of Conduct, Performance and Ethics for Nurses and Midwives* (NMC 2008a).
- As this is Dawn's final placement before registration the mentor must ensure that she has experienced effective professional and inter-professional working relationships to support learning for entry to the register.

9 What competencies/skills are transferable from this case study?

The competencies or transferable skills that are evident from this case study might include:

- **communication** – ability to communicate orally, in writing, or via electronic means, in a manner appropriate to the team;
- **teamwork** – being a constructive team member, contributing practically to the success of the team;
- **leadership** – being able to motivate and encourage others, whilst taking the lead;
- **initiative** – ability to see opportunities and to set and achieve goals;
- **problem solving** – thinking things through in a logical way in order to determine key issues, often also including creative thinking;
- **flexibility/adaptability** – ability to handle change and adapt to new situations;
- **self-awareness** – knowing your strengths and skills and having the confidence to put these across;
- **commitment/motivation** – having energy and enthusiasm in pursuing projects;
- **interpersonal skills** – ability to relate well to others and to establish good working relationships;
- **numeracy** – competence and understanding of numerical data, statistics and graphs.

Case Study 2
Standard: Facilitation of Learning

1 What are the key issues arising from this case study?

The student has learning needs in relation to the following:

- Exploring the integration of inter-professional working and learning in practice.
- Valuing and respecting the contribution of other members of the healthcare team.
- Her professional behaviour and attitude towards other healthcare professionals.
- Enabling her to complete her practice assessment successfully.

2 How could you as a mentor facilitate Joanne's learning needs during her placement?

The mentor has a professional responsibility to facilitate Joanne's learning needs and to provide appropriate learning opportunities to help her meet the required level of proficiency in her practice assessment. She could conduct an intermediate interview which explores Joanne's:

- communication skills;
- understanding of the incidents with the other members of the healthcare team;
- knowledge levels about the roles and contribution of other healthcare team members in providing a quality and seamless service;
- learning needs in order for her to achieve the required proficiency level in her practice assessment.

Following this:

- Devise an action plan with appropriate learning opportunities to meet Joanne's individual learning needs which are commensurate with her stage of training. This could involve spending time with other members of the healthcare team and allowing her to co-ordinate the care needs of clients which incorporate an inter-professional approach.
- Incorporate, as part of the action plan, weekly meetings which promote discussion and reflection upon Joanne's learning experiences.

3 What steps can you take as a mentor to ensure that your knowledge and practice on the facilitation of learning is current?

- Conduct a self-assessment of current abilities in relation to the NMC (2008b) standards and NHS KSF (DH 2004) around the subject of facilitating learning.
- Have discussions with the university link lecturer around curriculum developments and new ways of working and learning, for example, online resources.
- Explore with peers different approaches to the facilitation of students' learning and a coherent placement experience.

4 What steps can you take to ensure that Joanne's learning needs are facilitated in your absence?

Ensuring that other members of the ward team are aware of:

- Joanne's learning needs;
- the plan of action that has been devised;
- the requirements of the practice assessment document;
- the need to involve other members of the healthcare team;
- the arrangements to meet weekly.

Case Study 3
Standard: Assessment and Accountability

1 What are the key issues arising from this case study?

- There is inadequate mentorship support in place for James.
- The assessment process has not been followed.
- There is lack of evidence to support the professional judgements made and the documentation is inadequate.
- James's professional behaviour is inappropriate for a student nurse.
- James does not understand the differences between the professional role boundaries of a healthcare assistant and a student nurse.

2 Has James received a fair assessment?

No, James has not received a fair assessment because:

- The assessment process was not followed, i.e. no midpoint assessment was done.
- The assessment was not reliable as there was inconsistency in the mentor support throughout his placement.

- The summative records did not reflect an accurate account of James's assessment as no evidence was included to support the assessor's decisions.
- Appropriate feedback was not provided to James about his behaviour and there was insufficient time for him to practise and demonstrate completion of the NMC outcomes.

3 What are the requirements for a fair assessment?

The requirements for a fair assessment include the following:

- An educational environment is provided which has been audited as suitable for students.
- The student has access to a named mentor who will work with him or her.
- The student is supported through team mentorship.
- The student has preliminary, midpoint and final interviews conducted at set times during the practice placement experience.
- Local policies and procedures are adhered to in relation to practice assessment.
- Regular constructive feedback regarding the student's performance is provided verbally and recorded on the practice assessment document.
- Where areas of concern are identified, an action plan is developed to address these. The personal tutor should be involved in this process.

All documentation should be fully completed and supported with the appropriate evidence regarding judgements made. Supplementary evidence may be included, for example written testimonies from other members of the team.

4 What evidence should have been collected from this case study?

- Evidence from the team related to the following incidents: answering back, shouting at a patient, performing a procedure that is not commensurate with his stage of training.
- Evidence from the other qualified staff members, which could have been supplemented if a patient had chosen to complain.
- Documentary testimonies from the team specifying details of the incident, actions taken at the time and including relevant signatures, dates and times.
- All evidence should be contained within the practice placement document.

5 How could James's assessment have been formally documented?

- The assessment document should have clear entries for preliminary, intermediate and final interviews.
- Feedback on performance should be documented in a chronological order

supplemented by the above evidence and recording the student's comments and signature.

- Any action plans agreed relating to the achievement of the NMC outcomes arising from the identified incidents must be agreed by the student, mentor and personal teacher, and verified by all parties involved.
- All judgements made about students' performance must be documented, supported by the appropriate evidence and demonstrate that due process has been applied.

6 What rights has James in relation to this assessment?

He has the right to expect the following:

- Access to a named mentor and where appropriate team mentorship.
- An environment which is conducive to meeting his learning needs, commensurate with his level of proficiency and stage of training.
- Appropriately prepared and experienced mentors to work a minimum of two shifts with him per week throughout his placement allocation.
- Mentors who offer regular contact to reflect together on practice and progress, identify areas for development and who complete the assessment document.
- Trust and higher education institution (HEI) systems which exist to enable him to:
  - ➢ complain about the assessment process not being conducted correctly;
  - ➢ appeal against an unfair assessment;
  - ➢ have any complaint or appeal investigated in a fair and transparent manner in line with the higher education institution (HEI) policies.
- Access to the civil courts seeking a judicial review of the decisions and actions of the mentor.
- Compliance with the European Convention of Human Rights (Council of Europe 1950).

7 What are the legal and ethical implications for the mentor in relation to this case study?

- The mentor is accountable for decisions made related to student assessment.
- The mentor must be able to justify the assessment verbally and in writing.
- Giving an unduly low grade which cannot be defended could constitute a negligent act.
- The mentor can be liable if information is given negligently, which the student relies upon, and as a result of that information the student suffers harm.
- Mentors are accountable in relation to their contract of employment as they

are expected to act with reasonable care and skill. If they fail to do this, disciplinary action may be taken.
- Mentors must be objective in their assessment of the student. Personality conflicts that are allowed to influence assessment invalidate the assessment.
- Mentors must record information accurately in relation to name, location, grade, date, time of assessment, content of assessment, grade of achievement, comments of the assessor/s and action taken. All this information will enable the mentor to respond appropriately to any questions raised regarding the assessment.
- A mentor is subject to the duties under the Health and Safety Act 1974, section 7, in ensuring that reasonable care is taken of the student's health and safety, in order to assist the employer in complying with health and safety regulations (HSE 1974).

8 What should have been undertaken differently by the mentor and the ward team in relation to supporting and assessing James?

- His mentor (Susan) should have been supported by the other members of the team so that when she went off sick another team member could have picked up the assessment.
- The midpoint interview should have been conducted on time, with action plans agreed with the student and the personal teacher in relation to the areas which required improvement.
- All feedback should have been recorded on the practice assessment document in a chronological format supported by relevant evidence.
- All practice placement staff should be conversant with the higher education institution (HEI), Trust and professional body requirements in providing a fair assessment.

9 What quality assurance implications arise from this case study?

Staff development issues related to:

1 conducting a fair assessment;
2 legal, ethical and professional responsibilities of a mentor.

- The public must be protected from practitioners who have not met the required standard of proficiency to be entered on to the professional register.
- A robust system of team mentorship must be developed.
- The standards associated with the educational audit for the approval of practice placements must be adhered to.
- The practice placement policies and procedures must be adhered to.

Case Study 4
Standard: Evaluation of Learning

1 What are the main issues arising from this case study?

The overall rating for this placement could be regarded as fair only.

- There are six areas between 62 per cent and 69 per cent, ten areas between 70 per cent and 80 per cent and four areas over 80 per cent spanning Teaching, Learning and Assessment, Student Progression and Achievement, and Student Support.
- The areas which probably need focusing upon initially relate to those scores below 70 per cent and relate to the following standards:
  - Student Support:
    - ➢ **5.6** Students are introduced to their mentor/associate mentor within the first 24 hours of being on the placement
    - ➢ **5.9** Students remain supernumerary
    - ➢ **5.19** Students are made to feel welcome and part of the team.
  - Student Progression and Achievement:
    - ➢ **5.4** Learning needs are recognized and help is given with the learning outcomes/action plans
    - ➢ **5.20** Good communications exist to facilitate the delivery of care.
  - Teaching, Learning and Assessment:
    - ➢ **5.14** There are up-to-date learning resources (books, journals, articles, IT) available for student use.

2 Whose responsibility is it to resolve the issues arising from this evaluation?

The responsibility lies with the placement team, not solely the placement educational lead, to resolve these areas.

Other key academic support staff must be involved in addressing the issue, for example the university link lecturer from the higher education institution/s that you associate with, and possibly Trust training and development personnel.

3 What needs to be undertaken as a result of this evaluation?

The following should be done:

- A meeting should be set up with the placement team to discuss the findings. The university link lecturer and others (identified above) may also be invited.

- An action plan with key activities and specific timescales for achievement should be drawn up and is signed by the placement educational lead on behalf of the placement and also the university link lecturer.

4 What additional resources can you draw upon to support the changes you are suggesting/making in order to convince your peers?

- Quality assurance processes. Reference to documents relating to the NMC Standards, Trust audit documentation, practice placement policies/guidelines, and higher education institution processes should be accessed.
- Change management literature (see references in end list plus the links suggested in the answer to Question 6).
- Department of Health documentation such as *Placements in Focus: Guidance for Education in Practice for Health Care Professions* (DH 2001).
- Learning needs information, for example the Vark learning preferences questionnaire (Fleming 2001).
- The NMC *Standards to Support Learning and Assessment in Practice*, which can be accessed at http://www.nmc-uk.org.
- The *RCN Guidance Toolkit*, which can be accessed at http://www.rcn.org.uk/.

5 The student evaluation identified that some current practices need to change. What change management approach/theoretical model could you propose to the placement educational lead which might assist this process?

The following websites provide a range of approaches to bring about individual and organizational change. The theoretical models can be applied in any setting to address issues or problems which require change. The websites are:

- http://www.businessballs.com/;
- http://www.jiscinfonet.ac.uk/infokits/change-management;
- http://www.en.wikipedia.org/wiki/Change_management.

6 A culture needs to be created within the clinical area that embeds a commitment by all practitioners towards self and peer evaluation processes. What steps could be taken to achieve this?

The following could be considered:

- Review the elements in Question 4, and determine your current capabilities in relation to these areas.
- Utilize appropriate models in order to make judgements about personal and professional learning needs, for example appraisal tools, NHS KSF Framework (DH 2004) and the NMC Standards (NMC 2008b).

- Explore opportunities for peer discussions, for example, your own personal performance and developmental needs, team mentorship meetings, adverse incidents, student evaluations or feedback, audit action plans, current curriculum activities.
- Ward/team meetings could support peer development through discussions on:
  - ➤ student support mechanisms;
  - ➤ student progression and achievement issues;
  - ➤ teaching, learning and assessment issues.

Case Study 5
Standard: Creating an Environment for Learning

1 **What are the key issues arising from this case study?**

- Student evaluations have identified the need to improve the learning environment.
- The clinical area is functioning at full capacity in terms of student numbers. There are implications for the number of appropriately qualified mentors who are available to support students.
- The Nursing and Midwifery Council do not recognize associate mentors and there is a need to support other staff to become mentors.
- Whilst Staff Nurse Jones has been asked to examine strategies for improving the learning environment and produce a series of recommendations, this must involve the opinions of the ward staff and representatives from the higher education institution (HEI).

2 **What support and resources should Amy access to help her with this task?**

- She should be accessing and talking to the university link lecturer, who will be able to provide her with resources relating to mentorship, practice placement policies, procedures and standards. Key documents from the higher education institution (HEI), the NMC and other relevant parties should be accessed.
- She should also be accessing and talking to current students and colleagues in the clinical area.

Other resources available to Amy are as follows:

- The NMC has developed Standards to Support Learning and Assessment in practice that have outcomes for mentors, practice teachers and teachers. The standards take the form of a developmental framework. The outcomes for each role are identified as different stages within the framework. It is possible to enter or exit from the framework at any stage, and each stage is not dependent on having met the outcomes of a previous stage. The NMC has agreed mandatory requirements for each part of the register, which can be accessed at http://www.nmc-uk.org/aDisplayDocument.aspx?documentID=4368.

- All higher education institution (HEI) documentation that relates to student placements and practice assessments.

3 Why is it important that students are able to identify their own learning needs?

It is important for students to identify appropriate goals to enable them to develop personally and professionally in their current practice and for lifelong learning.

4 What processes exist to help students identify their learning needs and what is the mentor's role in relation to this?

- The Personal Development Planning (PDP) process for student nurses. Consult your university lead link for access to the documentation related to the HEI that you link with.
- Action plans can be used for both hub (main placement) and spoke (additional placement experiences which link to the speciality of the hub placement) placements and the retrieval of students who have been referred in practice.
- The mentor can develop spoke placements which support student learning and achievement of practice outcomes.
- The mentor can assist students to identify their own learning styles. There are various tools that enable a student to identify these. An example can be accessed at http://www.vark-learn.com/english/index.asp
- The mentor must know the student's stage of training and the outcomes expected at that stage and level. Please look at current student documentation and compare the descriptors for the different stages of training.
- The mentor must review the learning needs of students continuously during the placement experience.

5 Give four examples of learning resources that could be provided to support students and staff development in this clinical area?

The following could be considered:

- Orientation pack including:

➤ welcome letter;
➤ description of the care setting;
➤ names and contact details for key individuals;
➤ a reminder of the key stages of the placement;
➤ glossary of key terms that the student will encounter;
➤ orientation discussion form where the student could note his or her concerns or fears about the placement;
➤ relevant and current reading list.

- Resource file with current literature relevant to practice area.
- Clinical area policies, protocols and a philosophy, which are up to date and accessible.
- Student notice board.
- Adoption of the WORLD model. For more information on this please read Channell (2002).
- Development of spoke placements to support hub placement learning and practice outcomes.
- The *RCN Toolkit* (RCN 2007) and the DH 2001 document provide information on how to create an effective learning environment.

6 **How can Amy support the other staff on the ward to ensure that students' learning needs are effectively met in a safe environment?**

- Discuss with the staff their roles and responsibilities in supporting students.
- Provide opportunities for staff to discuss how students' learning needs can be best facilitated in the placement area.
- Encourage all staff to be actively involved in the updating and review of learning resources.
- Ensure practice polices and procedures are accessible for all staff and students.

7 **Why is it important for students to experience working with members of the multi-professional team?**

- To develop their understanding of the roles and responsibilities of the multi-professional team.

Further information about students working in a multidisciplinary team can be accessed from the DH (2001) website.

8 **How can Amy provide opportunities for inter-professional learning?**

- By providing spoke placements. Refer to your local higher education policy to read more about hub and spoke placements policies and guidelines.
- By encouraging attendance and participation in multidisciplinary team meetings.

- By encouraging engagement with other professionals in daily clinical practice.

9 **What strategies could Amy develop to continuously monitor the quality of the learning environment?**

- Regular meetings with university staff to discuss student evaluations and progress in relation to the audit action plan.
- Regular discussions with other members of the ward team and students about the quality of the learning environment.
- Self-evaluate the learning environment using the *RCN Toolkit* (RCN 2007) and *Placements in Focus* (DH 2001).

Case Study 6
Standard: Context of Practice

1 **What are the main issues arising from this case study?**

- Kelsey was not fully prepared to undertake the responsibility of caring for this patient.
- The delegated activity was not appropriate for her capabilities, stage of training and supernumerary status.
- The mentor is ultimately professionally accountable for the delegated activity.
- Kelsey did not ask for help when it was needed.
- Kelsey was not appropriately supervised throughout this procedure.
- The student is there to learn within the context of clinical practice, not to complete workload within limited staff resources.
- The appropriateness of the learning environment may need to be reviewed in the future if this incident was not an isolated problem.
- Patient safety and risk management issues from a clinical governance perspective need to be applied to the learning environment.
- There are a number of legal, ethical and professional issues here e.g. advocacy, patient assault, professional responsibilities under the *Code of Professional Conduct: Standards for Conduct, Performance and Ethics* (harm, risk, co-operation with others in the team, involvement of other carer(s) in the context of practice delivery).
- There was a complaint about the standard of care delivered.

2 **What does the context of practice in this case study suggest to you about the learning environment of this placement?**

- The context of care delivery may need to be reviewed in order to ensure safe and effective care.
- Specifically this relates to policies and guidelines regarding care delivery and student supervision and support in care delivery.
- The placement as a learning environment may need to be reviewed in relation to the suitability of student learning opportunities.
- Student supervision and support as a supernumerary learner, inter-professional learning and working and the standard and quality of care delivery will need to be reviewed.
- The relationship between the philosophy of care on the ward and actual practice may need to be considered.

RCN (2003) will help you review the philosophy of care to enable you to contextualize practice from this case study and explore the current approach adopted in your placement area.

3 Was Kelsey appropriately supervised?

No. The student was not appropriately supervised in this situation because:

- Her role as a student is as a learner, not a worker in clinical practice.
- Kelsey should have been supernumerary to the clinical workforce in her role as a learner.
- She had been delegated to care for three patients. It is unclear whether an assessment was undertaken by her mentor on:
    - ➢ her capabilities commensurate with her stage of training; and
    - ➢ the comments from her previous practice mentor about Kelsey having a quiet disposition and rarely asking questions.
- Kelsey was unaware of ward guidelines. It is unclear whether this was a problem with her lack of knowledge or whether the mentor had failed to inform her of these guidelines.

In order to supervise effectively mentors must:

- Have an accurate understanding of the Nursing and Midwifery Council's (NMC) position regarding student supernumerary status, accountability and responsibility.
- Be aware that the level of supervision required will vary according to the nature of the activity and the competence level of the student. This is articu-lated in the NMC (2008b) *Standard to Support Learning and Assessment in Practice*.
- Discuss supernumerary status and supervision with the student upon commencement of the placement to check that there is a common under-

standing of this requirement. Seek clarification from higher education institution (HEI) guidance regarding supernumerary status.
- Review the student's previous performance levels to determine future developmental needs.
- Maximize student learning in the clinical environment (see Channell 2002).

4 How could this situation have been prevented?

- By carrying out an initial assessment of Kelsey's capabilities.
- By ensuring appropriate supervision of Kelsey.
- By appropriate delegation of care.
- Kelsey could have requested assistance and support.
- Kelsey should have been made aware of ward guidelines, policies and procedures.
- By ensuring that inter-professional colleagues request assistance from appropriate staff.
- The mentor should be aware of what to do in the following situations:

  ➢ Giving feedback to the student.
  ➢ Documenting the discussion of the feedback with the student.
  ➢ Identifying future learning needs in line with her learning outcomes.
  ➢ Communicating with the personal tutor.
  ➢ Reflecting on the behaviour of the student in line with her assessment criteria.
  ➢ Reflecting on the role of the mentor in this situation.

5 How could the mentor have used the information from previous placements?

- By discussing Kelsey's learning needs at the preliminary assessment meeting.
- By identifying and discussing expectations with her.
- By checking her clinical skills record booklet on what has been achieved to date.

6 What are the legal and ethical implications for the mentor arising from this case study?

- Legal issues:

  ➢ The professional accountability of the mentor including the delegation of care activities to others.
  ➢ The duty of care owed to the patient and parent.
  ➢ The standard of care being given (there is the potential for litigation).

- Ethical issues:

➤ The lack of support demonstrated to the student and the parent.

➤ Undue pain and upset caused to the patient.

➤ The failure of the student to ask for help and articulate limitations.

➤ The failure by practitioners to act as an advocate for the patient.

7 **What different approaches could the mentor and the ward team take to improve the learning environment for students?**

- The philosophy of the learning environment could be evaluated.
- Ensure that inter-professional colleagues are aware of the role and status of students.
- Ensure practice guidelines and policies are easily accessible, discussed and applied by students and mentors.
- Ensure students are supernumerary in practice.
- Review with staff their approach to mentoring.
- Develop with staff a content list of items which should be discussed at student interviews.
- Promote evidence-based practice to ensure that it is used in everyday practice.

8 **How can the mentor address the inter-professional working relationship between student nurses and other healthcare professionals?**

- Identify the inter-professional team and their specific roles within the clinical area.
- Develop and facilitate spoke placements with relevant healthcare professionals.
- Encourage students to identify inter-professional working as a learning need whilst on placement.
- Involve students in inter-professional meetings and teaching sessions.

Case Study 7
Standard: Evidence-based Practice

1 **How would you plan to support Josie's learning to facilitate the meeting of the development need identified in her personal development portfolio?**

- By assessing her current level of knowledge in relation to how research is used to influence patient care.
- Develop a plan of action for her to look at Trust policies, protocols, local

and national guidelines and pathways relevant to the area of practice and identify how these are informed by evidence.

- Encourage Josie to identify mechanisms within the Trust for agreeing policies and protocols.
- As part of a spoke placement Josie could visit the audit department and discuss how audit processes influence local practices.
- Direct Josie to relevant sources of information (see 'Possible sources of materials to inform your knowledge and practice', pages 83–85.
- Provide an opportunity for a discussion to evaluate what she has learned.
- Discuss with Josie how research articles can be assessed using the CASP model (PHRU 2007) to determine the quality of the study and if the findings/ recommendations should be implemented.

2 How can you encourage Josie to inform herself in relation to evidence-based practice?

- Encourage her to utilize ward/Trust resources e.g. journals, books, learning packs, personnel (e.g. specialist nurses and patients), the library, the audit department and the Research and Development department.
- Direct Josie to online resources, health organization websites (e.g. NICE) and databases (e.g. CINAHL Medline, Cochrane).
- By suggesting other reading in this subject area. Please see the list of reading materials/contacts that are provided on pages 83–85.

3 How would you assess Josie's competency to provide a rationale based on best evidence to justify safe nursing practice?

- By the quality of the sources she uses e.g. peer-reviewed journal articles, research, reputable organizations.
- The sources she uses should be up to date.
- She should show some ability to appraise the evidence and judge its worth.

4 How would you assess Josie's competency at questioning nursing practice in terms of its evidence base?

- By looking at her ability to reflect upon particular care delivery activities carried out in a span of duty.
- By assessing whether she can identify evidence in relation to specific activities.
- By judging her ability at questioning issues around the quality of care delivered (effectiveness of intervention and possibly costs via the resources used).
- By exploring how she distinguishes between different levels of evidence such as randomized control trials, locally agreed practices and anecdotal evidence.

5 How would you assess Josie's ability to search for new evidence which may have an impact upon patient care?

• Ask Josie to identify an aspect of care and then ask her to provide evidence from a range of sources which may inform that aspect. This should include her ability to provide evidence from electronic and local resources (e.g. protocols, pathways, policies etc.).
• You need to establish the processes she adopts to search for evidence and the analytical steps used to judge the information collected.
• Discuss how decisions are made about nursing interventions which draw upon this evidence and the views of the patient.

6 What are the professional and ethical implications for the mentor and the student in relation to this case study?

• Requirements of the NMC *Code of Professional Conduct: Standards for Conduct, Performance and Ethics* (NMC 2008) in relation to being up to date and utilizing best evidence to support practice.
• A breach of the Code could result in unfitness for practice and harm to the patient.
• Nonmaleficence: the nurse must do the patient no harm.
• The NMC *Code of Professional Conduct: Standards for Conduct, Performance and Ethics* (NMC 2008) requires the nurse to treat people as individuals, promote advocacy and respond to concerns and preferences.

7 Are there any implications for the Trust, the higher education institution and the public arising out of this case study?

• Compliance must occur with their policies and protocols.
• Care may not be based on best evidence, undermining the faith and trust the public place in the healthcare provider.
• Practice placements should explore ways of increasing/reviewing the evidence base to support practice e.g. journal clubs, resources such as journals, books, learning packs, electronic tools etc.

Case Study 8
Standard: Leadership

1 At what level does leadership take place in an organization and specifically on Braxton ward? Using the leadership standards of the NMC as guidelines, identify whether leadership has failed in this instance?

• Leadership takes place at all levels of the organization. Corporate vision and values play a central role in an organization's strategic planning, its management and key activities. For example:

> ➤ Vision: Where are we going?
> ➤ Mission: How are we going to get there?
> ➤ Values: How do we need to be to get there?

- Understanding and sharing their organization's vision, mission and values helps staff to be clear about the purpose of their work at every level and how it contributes to the wider organizational goals.
- Ward managers and placement educational leads are responsible for leadership issues at ward level. Using the new NMC Standards previously listed under the leadership requirements, they must ensure and 'demonstrate leadership skills for education within practice and academic settings' and can empower staff by involving them in the creation of a ward or departmental vision and the means to achieve it.
- In this instance, the vision, mission and values in terms of the NMC requirements for leadership have not been met and this can be identified if a comparison is made between what happened on the ward and the provided standards.

2 **What are the major elements of leadership and how does this link to the role of the placement educational lead and mentor in this case study?**

- Being an effective leader is essentially about having and communicating a vision and empowering others to achieve it. In this case the vision is related to achieving the NMC standards in demonstrating leadership skills in education and practice.
- Effective leaders know when they are likely to be overstretched and must delegate to staff. The delegation of tasks is a key way of developing and motivating staff.
- Whilst the student has been allocated a mentor, George as ward manager should have been aware of the student's special circumstances during the process of the induction to the ward and the identification of the student's needs.
- He was aware that Vivian had gone off sick and should have briefed Albert Stokes that he would be consulting him on the student's progress and the need to involve him in the final assessment.
- It must be understood that only qualified mentors are responsible for signing the documentation.
- To delegate successfully, time must be taken to brief staff properly and explain what their objectives and tasks are.
- A good leader must monitor and provide on a regular basis but not to the extent of undermining the delegate's autonomy.
- George should have checked periodically with Albert that all was well and spoken to the student himself.

- When a member of staff has completed a delegated task, a good leader should work with that person to identify any lessons that can be learnt for the future. George could have used Albert's supervision of the student as a learning opportunity.
- A good leader should meet with staff on a regular basis to review and discuss:
  - ➢ progress made towards achieving objectives;
  - ➢ deviations from plans;
  - ➢ problems or issues requiring non-urgent decisions;
  - ➢ possible improvements in processes and systems.
- It would appear that communication was an issue on the ward. George also has two willing candidates for the mentorship module and should make the applications a priority.

3 Who, in this case study, was and wasn't exercising leadership in relation to this student?

- Remind yourself again of the NMC requirements for leadership as any comments in relation to the lack of implementation of the above standards are relevant.
- George was not an effective leader at ward level. There was a lack of understanding on his part as to what is required under the NMC standards (NMC 2008b). In fact, George did not manage either in this case study.
- There was poor delegation and it appears that the ward staff were not clear about their role.
- Poor team spirit, low morale and also a lack of support for him in his new role may have contributed to George's failure to demonstrate effective leadership.
- There is a desire among staff to progress and undertake the degree mentorship module, but George's poor time management in organizing the resources to fund this development is a matter of concern.
- There is a failure of advocacy in relation to identifying students' learning opportunities and planning their learning experiences.

4 What do you think George's priorities should have been?

- George should have checked that the student had met with his mentor on commencement to the ward and that specific learning needs were identified.
- George should know whether appropriate learning opportunities were organized to meet the student's individual needs.
- It could be that he did reallocate the student to Albert when Vivian went off sick (although this may have been the case, we have not been told) but knew that Albert could not sign any of the documentation as he is not a registered mentor.

- At this stage George should have checked with Albert that he understood the situation, had a remedial plan and would be involved in the final assessment. George's role would involve regular communication and support for Albert.
- George could also have involved the rest of the ward team in helping the student progress and obtain feedback from them as well.
- Alternatively, George could have taken on the mentor role himself. He should not have refused to sign the documentation but consulted with his staff as to the student's progress.
- The above comments refer to delegation of role. Effective leaders know when they are likely to be overstretched and must delegate to staff. The delegation of tasks is a key way of developing and motivating staff. To delegate successfully:

  ➤ Take the time to brief staff properly and explain what their objectives and tasks are.
  ➤ Monitor and provide support and advice on a regular basis but not to the extent that you undermine the delegate's autonomy.
  ➤ After a member of staff has completed a delegated task, work with them to identify any lessons that can be learnt for the future.

5 **What actions should be undertaken at the organizational and individual level to address this case study?**

- George, as ward manager, in the absence of a placement educational lead, is ultimately responsible for student placements on his ward. George appears not to be coping with his ward manager role. Perhaps students should be removed from the ward until the ward problems have been sorted out. Think about this.
- Regular ward meetings could be introduced to establish what the problems are and to develop a new team spirit. The delegation of tasks is a key way of developing and motivating staff.
- The continuing professional development needs of staff should be established and applications implemented by George.
- Albert and John should insist that they undertake the mentorship programme, as there is a clear need for more staff to be involved in supervising students.
- In the interim, it could be that Albert and John, whilst waiting to commence a mentor module, could attend an associate mentor workshop. This would be a temporary measure, but might alleviate some of the pressure on George.
- George could request a meeting with the university link lecturer responsible for student placements on the ward to review the learning opportunities and develop the learning environment on the ward.

Case Study 9
Group Assessment Exercise

1 What are the key issues arising from this case study?

- This is her final week and the student's final interview is due as part of her summative assessment and there is no retrieval time for developing an action plan to overcome this.
- The student has not achieved some of the proficiencies expected at this stage of her training.
- It could be interpreted that the mentor failed to pick this up earlier in the placement or the opportunity never arose until the last week of placement experience.
- The mentor cannot use the recent disclosure of the student's dyslexia to alter the outcome of the assessment process.
- The mentor needs to take action now.
- The student will need reassurance.

2 What actions should the mentor take?

- Check if any of the other mentors/associate mentors had identified that the student demonstrated difficulties with documentation.
- Collect all evidence which indicates that the student has difficulties with documenting care.
- Inform the student verbally and in writing on her assessment document that she has not achieved the required standard of proficiency in her practice assessment (in one or more domains/proficiencies).
- Justify the reasons for her decisions objectively, both verbally and in writing.
- Contact the student's personal tutor as soon as possible to arrange an urgent meeting between the mentor, the student and the personal tutor to discuss the assessment decision.
- Advise the student to reflect upon the communications and the decision which has been taken, and suggest that she might wish to consider her response in preparation for the joint meeting with the mentor and personal tutor.

3 Are there any practice placement resources which would help the mentor in this situation?

See for example:

- *The Code: Standards of Conduct, Performance and Ethics for Nurses and midwives* (NMC 2008b).

- Guidelines for dealing with student issues in clinical placement.
- Practice placement policies for pre-registration undergraduate programmes.
- The procedure for completing the practice placement assessment document.

4 What do you think are the needs of the student here?

- The student needs to be commended for disclosing her dyslexia and reassured that now the problem has been identified appropriate help and support can be given.
- The student should be made aware of any available dyslexia resources.
- The student should be fully informed of all the decisions and actions taken to date.
- The student should be treated fairly in respect of her assessment and provided with the opportunities and support to retrieve her failure.
- She should be offered the opportunity to contact her personal tutor or other contacts for support.

5 What are the professional responsibilities for the mentor in this situation?

- To adhere to the NMC requirements under *the Code of Professional Conduct: Standards for Conduct, Performance and Ethics* (NMC 2008b) as she is accountable for the decisions and actions taken in relation to this student assessment.
- To protect the public from practitioners who have not met the required standard of proficiency to be entered on to the professional register.
- To manage the 'failing student' so that she may either enhance her performance and capabilities or be able to understand her failure and the implications of this for future practice.
- To be accountable in relation to her contract of employment as she will be expected to act with reasonable care and skill in the performance of her duties as a mentor.
- To record all information accurately in relation to the student assessment, including the decision taken, the supportive evidence, all communications with the student and actions taken such as contacting the personal tutor.

References

BusinessBalls.com (1995–2010) *Ethical Work and Life Learning.* http://www.businessballs.com/ (Accessed 25 February 2010).
Channell, W. (2002) Helping students to learn in the clinical environment, *Nursing Times*, 98(39): 34–5.

Council of Europe (1950) *European Convention of Human Rights.* http://www.hri.org/docs/ECHR50.html (Accessed 25 February 2010).

DH (Department of Health) (2001) *Placements in Focus. Guidance for Education in Practice for Health Care Professions.* http://www.dh.gov.uk/en/Publicationsandstatistics/Publications/PublicationsPolicyAndGuidance/DH_4009511 (Accessed 25 February 2010).

DH (2004) *The NHS Knowledge and Skills Framework (NHS KSF) and the Development Review Process.* http://www.rcn.org.uk/__data/assets/pdf_file/0004/270544/003550.pdf (Accessed 25 February 2010).

Fleming, N. (2001) *Teaching and Learning Styles: VARK Strategies.* http://www. vark-learn.com/english/index.asp (Accessed 25 February 2010).

HSE (Health and Safety Executive) (1974) *The Health and Safety at Work etc Act.* http://www.hse.gov.uk/legislation/hswa.htm (Accessed 15 February 2010).

Jisc Infonet (2009) *Change Management.* http://www.jiscinfonet.ac.uk/infokits/change-management (Accessed 25 February 2010).

NMC (Nursing and Midwifery Council) (2008a) *The Code: Standards of Conduct, Performance and Ethics for Nurses and Midwives.* http://www.nmc-uk.org/aArticle.aspx?ArticleID=3056 (Accessed 25 February 2001).

NMC (2008b) *Standards to Support Learning and Assessment in Practice.* http://www.nmc-uk.org/aDisplayDocument.aspx?documentID=4368 (Accessed 25 February 2010).

PHRU (2007) *CASP Appraisal Tools.* http://www.phru.nhs.uk/Pages/PHD/resources.htm (Accessed 25 February 2010).

RCN (Royal College of Nursing) (2003) *Children and Young People's Nursing: A Philosophy of Care. Guidance for Nursing Staff.* http://www.rcn.org.uk/__data/assets/pdf_file/0003/78573/002012.pdf (Accessed 25 February 2010).

RCN (2007) *RCN Guidance for Mentors of Nursing Students and Midwives: An RCN Toolkit.* http://www.rcn.org.uk/__data/assets/pdf_file/0008/78677/002797.pdf (Accessed 25 February 2010).

Wikipedia (2010) *Change Management.* http://www.en.wikipedia.org/wiki/Change_management (Accessed 25 February 2010).

Glossary

Accountability: Accountability in nursing is an integral part of professional practice since, in the course of that practice, the practitioner has to make judgements in a wide variety of circumstances and be answerable for those judgements.

Annual updating: The NMC requires mentors to provide evidence of an annual update which is a requirement for maintaining ongoing competence in fulfilling this professional role. Annual updating can be undertaken in a variety of ways. Here are a few exemplars:

1 Attendance at and associated reflection on mentor development study days or similar organized activities.
2 Participation in mentor support forums, or other working groups related to mentor learning and development.
3 Personal development activities which may include researching and reflecting upon an educational topic and/or working with other experts/ role models.
4 Participating in a group meeting with peers to discuss the validity and reliability of judgements made during an assessment in challenging situations.

Associate mentor: A qualified member of staff who works under the guidance of the mentor in the supervision, teaching and facilitation of students. This is predominantly a local Greater Manchester term which is not recognized nationally for those practitioners who are involved with mentors in the teaching and learning process.

Bolam test: This is a measure of whether the doctor has discharged his or her standard of care in the management of the patient.

Case study: A case study is an in-depth investigation/study of a single individual, group, incident, or community. Rather than using samples and following a rigid protocol to examine a limited number of variables, case study methods involve an in-depth, longitudinal examination of a single instance or event: a case.

Continuing personal development (CPD): This is the term that describes a commitment to structured skills enhancement and personal or professional competence.

Core dimensions: The NHS KSF is made up of 30 dimensions. The dimensions identify broad functions that are required by the NHS to enable it to provide a good quality service to the public. Six of the dimensions are core, which means that they are relevant to every post in the NHS. The core dimensions are: 1 Communication 2 Personal and People Development 3 Health, Safety and Security 4 Service Improvement 5 Quality 6 Equality and Diversity. http://www.rose.nhs.uk/SiteCollectionDocuments/NHS_KSF.doc (Accessed 22 December 2009).

Employer-led development review: The NHS Knowledge and Skills Framework (NHS KSF) and the Development Review Process. The development review is a partnership process undertaken between an individual member of staff and a reviewer. The reviewer will usually be the individual's line manager but the role can also be delegated to someone else. If the reviewer role is delegated, then the individual to whom it is delegated will need to be competent to act in that role and also have sufficient authority to be able to arrange learning and development opportunities. Many reviewers will need support to develop their knowledge and skills in this area; they will also need to commit sufficient time to undertake the development review process effectively as it will become a key feature of ongoing NHS work. http://www.rdash.nhs.uk/wp-content/uploads/2009/11/Performance-and-Development-Review.pdf (Accessed 22 December 2009).

Evidence: In its broadest sense this includes everything that is used to determine or demonstrate the truth of an assertion.

Evidence-based practice: This is an approach to healthcare in which evidence is sought to underpin best practice.

Feedback: This describes the situation when output from (or information about the result of) an event in the past will influence the same event in the present or future. When an event is part of a chain of cause and effect that forms a circuit or loop, then the event is said to 'feed back' into itself.

Fitness for practice: The NMC safeguards the public through controlling entry to and maintenance of the register. Above all, public protection is achieved through a process of professional self-regulation that ensures fitness to practice. It upholds professional standards and protects the public; it requires all practitioners to recognize what is acceptable and unacceptable practice; it demands that all employees work in the best interests of the public. http://www.nmc-uk.org/aFrameDisplay.aspx?DocumentID=768 (Accessed 22 December 2009).

Framework to Support Learning and Assessment in Practice: In August 2006 the NMC published standards to support learning and assessment in practice, reflecting the responses to consultations, and the final standards approved by Council in March 2006. The standards replaced those previously published for the preparation of teachers of nurses, midwives and specialist community public health nurses (NMC 2004) and included new standards for mentors and practice teachers. NMC Circular 17/2007 made explicit the requirement for programme and placement providers to implement the standards, which have been mandatory since 1 September 2007. This included the requirement for mentor, practice teacher and teacher programmes to have gained NMC approval prior to accepting students on to such programmes from 1 September 2007. http://www.nmc-uk.org/ aDisplayDocument.aspx?documentID=4368 (Accessed 22 December 2009).

Higher education institution: The university that delivers the pre- and post-qualifying registration programmes and works in partnership with healthcare providers to place students on clinical placements.

Inter-professional learning: The 'occasions when two or more professions learn with, from and about each other to improve collaboration and the quality of care' (Caipe 2005). Inter-professional learning enables different health and social care workers and agencies to gain a greater appreciation of each other's values, knowledge and abilities and facilitates the best use of their skills.

Knowledge and skills framework (KSF): The KSF defines and describes the knowledge and skills which NHS staff (except doctors and dentists) need to apply in their work in order to deliver quality services. It provides a single, consistent, comprehensive and explicit framework on which review and development of all staff is based. http://www.scqf.org.uk/nmsruntime/ saveasdialog.aspx?lID=139&sID (Accessed 22 December 2009).

KSF and associated personal development planning and review (PDPR) process: A process which helps to ensure that staff are supported to be effective in their jobs and committed to developing and maintaining high quality service for the public.

Live register: The NMC (2008) states that placement providers are responsible for ensuring that 'an up-to-date local register of current mentors and practice teachers is held and maintained.' This register must be regularly reviewed and kept updated with registrants' names being added or removed as necessary.

Local register: The NMC requires practice placement providers to keep and maintain up-to-date local registers of mentors and processes for the review and maintenance of mentor qualifications including annual updating and triennial review. This should also include information about mentors' initial qualifications, mentor qualification and date of mentor updates attended.

Mandatory: Required or commanded by authority; obligatory.

Mentor: A registered nurse who has met the outcomes of the NMC (2008) standards to 'support learning and assessment in practice'.

NHS KSF development review process: The development review is a partnership process undertaken between an individual member of staff and 'a reviewer'. The reviewer will usually be the individual's line manager but the role can also be delegated to someone else. If the reviewer role is delegated, then the individual to whom it is delegated will need to be competent to act in that role and also have sufficient authority to be able to arrange learning and development opportunities. Many reviewers will need support to develop their knowledge and skills in this area; they will also need to commit sufficient time to undertake the development review process effectively as it will become a key feature of ongoing NHS work. http://www.unison.org.uk/acrobat/B1961.pdf (Accessed 22 December 2009).

NMC Standard: The standard takes the form of a developmental framework with specific outcomes for mentors, practice teachers and teachers. The framework defines and describes the knowledge and skills nurses and midwives need to apply in practice when they support and assess students on NMC approved programmes which lead to a recordable qualification on the NMC register. The NMC have agreed mandatory requirements for each part of the register. The outcomes for each role are identified as different stages within the framework. http://www.easterngp.co.uk/page.php?page_id=432 (Accessed 22 December 2009).

Peer evaluation: The process of checking another's work against the requirements that have been given and giving constructive feedback.

Performance criteria: The standards by which student performance is evaluated. Performance criteria help assessors maintain objectivity and provide students with important information about expectations, giving them a target or goal to strive for.

Personal development plan (PDP): A personal development plan identifies the individual's learning and development needs and interests and how these will be taken forward. The PDP is the outcome of the planning stage of the development review process. Within the National Agreement, there is a commitment on both sides – managers and individual members of staff – to the achievement of PDPs within agreed time periods, usually by the next review date. http://www.telford.nhs.uk/Staff-Zone/Learning-Opportunities/KSF-and-e-KSF/KSF-Overview/ (Accessed 22 December 2009).

Placement educational lead: The placement educational lead is the responsibility of the ward manager but the main functions of the role may be delegated to another senior member of staff within the placement area. The placement educational lead will work in partnership with clinical and educational colleagues to help the development of an effective learning environment within the placement area.

Practice placement provider: The practice placement provider is the organization where students complete their clinical placements. Practice placement providers have specific responsibilities related to the maintenance of clinical placements and the mentor register.

Professional development portfolio: A professional tool to help nurses record their career and post-registration education and practice. It provides a clear and concise framework within which a comprehensive resource can be built up that will be useful in a variety of ways, including: applying for a new post; compiling a CV; seeking accreditation for prior learning and experience; participating in performance review; building a personal development profile; and meeting the statutory requirements for renewing NMC registration. http://www.whsmith.co.uk/CatalogAndSearch/ProductDetails.aspx?productID=9780443074332 (Accessed 1 March 2010).

Reductionist: The analysis of something into simpler parts or organized systems, especially with a view to explaining or understanding it.

Registrant: A registered nurse who has met the standards of proficiency for nurse registration nurse education and has been declared as being of good health and good character. Each practitioner must work within the NMC Code, meet the Post Registration and Practice (PREP) standards, complete a notification of practice form and pay the annual renewal fee.

Reliability: This refers to the consistency with which a test measures what it is designed to measure. If a test is deemed to be reliable the results would be the same if the test were to be reapplied at a different time to the same student(s).

Reviewer/Appraiser: A mentor in practice will be appraised by a named reviewer. The reviewer may be a direct line manager or, alternatively, a named individual who has been delegated this responsibility by his or her direct line manager.

Self-evaluation: The evaluation by self against goals, objectives and performance methods.

Sign-off mentors: These are nurses who make judgements about whether a student has met the standards of proficiency for entry to the professional register or a qualification that is recorded on the NMC register. Sign-off mentors will have to be on the same part or sub-part on which the student is intending to register and working in the same field of practice e.g. adult, child etc. To become a sign-off mentor the Nursing and Midwifery Council have identified additional criteria in the *Standards to Support Learning and Assessment in Practice* (NMC 2008: Section 2.1.3), which all nurse mentors must undertake.

Transferable: Learning that can be transferred from one context to similar situations.

Triennial review: In a triennial review, which takes place once every three years, employers will be expected to undertake a review of an individual's performance as a mentor. Placement providers can decide the format of a triennial review of mentors but it may form part of an employer-led development appraisal. http://www.nmc-uk.org/aFrameDisplay.aspx?Document ID=4368 (Accessed 22 December 2009).

Validity: This is the extent upon which a test measures what it is designed to measure. If an assessment is unreliable then it lacks validity as it may produce the same results every time but not measure what it is intended to measure. Validity can be broken down into a number of categories such as face validity, construct validity, content validity, concurrent validity and predictive validity. To infer validity involves the collection of evidence of these different categories in relation to the test or assessment being carried out in clinical practice.

Workshop: An educational seminar or series of meetings emphasizing interaction and exchange of information among a usually small number of participants.

References

CAIPE (Centre for the Advancement of Interprofessional Education) (2002) http://www.caipe.org.uk/about-us/defining-ipe/ (Accessed 25 February 2010).

NMC (Nursing and Midwifery Council) (2004) *Standards for the Preparation of Teachers of Nurses, Midwives and Specialist Community Public Health Nurses*. London: NMC.

NMC (2008) *Standards to Support Learning and Assessment in Practice: NMC Standards for Mentors, Practice Teachers and Teachers*. London: NMC.

Index